A Need for Living

Signposts on the journey of life and beyond

Tom Gordon

Chaplain
Marie Curie Centre, Fairmile
Edinburgh

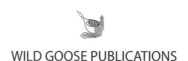

WILD GOOSE PUBLICATIONS

A Need for Living

Contents

Dedication

To Mary, Mairi, Kathryn and James,
for being the unique individuals they are,
and for all the love and laughter we share as a family

Acknowledgements

I can't write an acknowledgement for this book without using one of my pictures. Writing a book is like giving birth. The gestation period during which the idea grows and the writing takes shape is long and often arduous, and is especially trying when it comes close to 'full term'. Then, when the child is born, through a time of difficult labour, there is your baby, complete, new, and amazing to behold. What follows is a sense of wonder – how did you get from the moment of conception all that time ago to this final product? And then comes what is, perhaps, the most scary part – you have to let it go, to see your creation take its own life, independent of you, with no idea what kind of existence it will have.

So, in watching and wondering how this child of mine will develop, I pause and rest after this birthing process to recall with gratitude those who have helped nurture 'my baby' to this stage. Thanks are due to Tom Paxton and Cherry Lane Music for their permission to quote one of Tom's songs and for giving me the title of the book; to all those people who know how important their encouragement has been with this project and many other facets of ministry over the years; to my good friend Dorothy Innes, Centre Director at the Marie Curie Centre Fairmile for twenty years, and to all my colleagues on the staff for their unfailing support and cooperation; to Sandra, Alex and the staff at Wild Goose Publications for their positive and affirming attitude, and for the suggestions and guidance which have made this a better book than I could have produced myself; for good friends and wise counsellors from whom I have gained insights, with whom I have shared love, and who have given me, often unwittingly, some of the images this book contains; and, most importantly, to my family, including those to whom this book is dedicated, for their love, enthusiasm, tolerance and good humour, and for always keeping my feet on the ground.

Finally, I pay tribute to those people who have allowed me to share their journey of life and faith, and who have welcomed me into personal and painful parts of their lives. There are those whose stories I tell in this book – and whose names and circumstances have been sufficiently altered to protect their anonymity – and those countless others with whom I have had the privilege to journey. For their willingness to trust and share, and for giving me much more than I have given them, I will be eternally grateful.

August 2001, Edinburgh

Introduction

Through all the changing scenes of life
Nahum Tate

Praying for grace, and faced with a need for living
Tom Paxton: Pandora's Box

Telling people at parties that I work in a hospice, and more espe-cially that I am a hospice chaplain, is a certain conversation-stopper. There are a number of standard reactions. Faces fall and take on a worried frown, voices which were light and cheerful become serious and heavy. And among the stock responses is the phrase: 'Goodness, that must be very depressing.'

I've thought a lot about that comment and my reaction – along the lines of: 'No, never depressing. Hard work, certainly. Stressful and sad at times? Yes, that too. But depressing? Never!' And why? Because my work, while perceived, not surprisingly, to be about dying, is in practice about living. And the people I work with – patients, carers and colleagues – are people who wish to live full lives even when faced with the reality of death.

I'm an enthusiast for what I do. I love my work! The satisfaction which comes from helping people deal with the important things of life in the face of death is very real and sustaining for me. And that is primarily because working in a hospice *is* about life in all its variety and changing scenes.

There's a Tom Paxton song called 'Pandora's Box' which contains these words:

> *Night passed so slowly, all the dreams were bad;*
> *Pandora's box fell down, it broke open.*
> *All of my memories – bound to make me sad –*

I heard every unkind word I'd spoken.
Hard though I tried, I couldn't get myself awake;
Hard though I cried, I would remember each mistake.
Praying for sunrise, prayers were all I had,
Prayers and all the promises I'd broken.

How can I make it, feeling this way,
Not at all convinced to go on living.
No place to go to, no excuse to stay,
One more soul in bad need of forgiving.
Hard though I tried, I couldn't get myself awake;
Hard though I cried, I would remember each mistake.
Hanging on 'til sunrise, living day by day,
Praying for grace, and faced with a need for living.

It is often only in the face of your own mortality that Pandora's box breaks open, and the jumble of memories and fears, mistakes and broken promises tumbles out and threatens to overwhelm you and destroy any sense of the rightness in living you had worked out along the way. So it is at that point that life has to be tackled in all its complexity. It is at that point that we hear the cry for grace, for meaning and purpose in the knowledge of the impermanence of life. And it is at that point that the chaplain's role in a hospice is real – when, faced with a need for living, people crave encouragement to live and to understand the fullness of their living, until they die.

This is the *raison d'être* for my work, and why I can say at parties I love what I do when others would consider it depressing. 'Faced with a need for living.' How can you fail to find satisfaction when your role is to help people with that?

What follows in these chapters, therefore, is a collection of reflections on pictures and people in the field of spiritual care, offering practical guidance for anyone's life journey when they seek meaning and purpose in living. You will be introduced to people who have been helped to live until they die, or to live through bereavement when they felt it was never going to be possible, or to live with illness and suffering and problems which threatened to overwhelm them completely. And you will hear some of the stories and be introduced to some of the images and techniques I have offered over the years to help them face their need for living. It is not an exhaustive account of my time as a hospice chaplain, since there are many more people whose stories could be told and, I am sure, many more pictures which, when formed and utilised, will continue to provide benefit to such people. Nor is it a textbook on chaplaincy or spiritual care, although I hope that there might be something in these reflections which will be helpful to readers in their personal search and professional practice. But it is an offering of a reflective process, one I myself have enjoyed and been stimulated by, and which I hope will be of use to others.

I hope that through meeting these people, reading these stories and reflections, and perhaps through your working with and thinking about the images which are contained in these chapters, you might come to understand why I say at parties that I enjoy the job I do and do not find it depressing. It is simply because when people are 'faced with a need for living' and are allowed to explore what that means, there is much living for them – and for me – in all its fullness and wonder, to be found and enjoyed.

Night thoughts

Night passed,
every moment an age,
every thought a fear,
every shadow a threat.
Night passed
so slowly.
God of the night,
be the God of my night
and leave me not alone.

Dreams came,
every image a memory,
every scene a question,
every wakening an emptiness,
leaving no peace.
God of the dreams,
be the God of my dreaming
and give me peace.

Memories came,
every remembrance a lifetime,
every mistake a burden,
every broken promise a cross

to cause me pain.
God of the memories
be the God of my memories
so I might remember you.

Prayers came,
every prayer a cry,
every plea with tears,
every intercession with longing
for a listening ear.
God of the prayers,
be the God of my prayers,
and listen.

Sunrise came,
every glimmer a hope,
every stirring a promise,
every desire a grace
for a new day.
God of the sunrise,
make your sun to rise for me now
in my need for living.

One

Preparing the paintings

Look here, upon this picture, and on this
William Shakespeare: Hamlet

The painted veil which those who live call Life
Percy Bysshe Shelley: Sonnet

There is a 'Peanuts' cartoon by the late Charles Schultz which depicts three small children, Lucy, Charlie Brown and Linus, lying on the pitcher's mound of a baseball park staring up into the sky. 'What do you see in the clouds, Linus?' enquires Lucy. 'Well,' replies her friend, 'over there I see an outline of the map of British Honduras in the Caribbean, and there I see the profile of Thomas Eakins the famous sculptor and artist, and further over I see the stoning of Stephen, and there is St Paul standing at the side.' 'And what do *you* see in the clouds, Charlie Brown?' Lucy asks. To which a forlorn Charlie Brown replies, 'Well, actually, I was *going* to say I see a Duckie and a Horsie, but I don't think I'll bother any more!'

The meaning is clear. Of *course* we see things differently. We can look at the same clouds and see different pictures, because we look at the same sky through different eyes, from different places, and with different experiences which determine our interpretation.

The problem Charlie Brown had is that what he saw in the clouds did not seem as impressive as the complicated picture Linus saw, and somehow, therefore, it seemed to him to be inferior, unworthy of further exploration. 'I don't think I'll bother any more.' It is the self-same problem we have with the different ways we see and interpret life's experiences. Of course we see things differently, because we are different people. We look into the same sky and see different things.

But when someone sees a picture with such clarity and with levels of complex interpretation at which we can only marvel, when we are only at the 'duckie' and 'horsie' stage, no wonder we feel we have missed out somewhere.

This is exactly the issue which I face in my work as a hospice chaplain. In the field of spiritual care, in explorations of the spiritual meaning of current experiences – especially in the face of death – people do see things differently. They express things differently. They interpret things differently. They are aware of the different patterns in 'the painted veil which those who live call life'. They find different pictures in the clouds.

So there is often a pressure, real or conceived – particularly among religious people and especially from a Christian perspective – to define the picture in one form for everyone, to 'standardise' the view so that one interpretation is acceptable and workable for all people and every circumstance. There is, therefore, the implication that one picture is right and the others are wrong. And there is the further tendency to make people feel that if their picture does not match up to this complicated, detailed standard, then they have somehow failed to grasp the truth of the real pattern in the clouds. Their interpretation is flawed – the Charlie Brown 'duckie and horsie' syndrome!

It is the task of those of us who work in the area of spiritual care to help people find, interpret and express the meaning of the picture they see. It is the task of those of us who work with dying and bereaved people to affirm that the duckie and horsie pictures are valid. It is our task to challenge those who would want to impose their own pictures and interpretations because that is what they see or have come to understand.

Part of my role as a chaplain is to 'demythologise' the field of spiritual care so that those who see what they see are not made to feel inferior to those who see things differently. This book is offered as part of this demythologising process. It arises from the challenges to my own thinking which I have had to face, and subsequent reinterpretations of some of the pictures I myself see in the clouds. It draws upon incidents in my work and reflections on people I have worked with who have taught me much from their 'duckie and horsie' point of view. It is an offering from my own continued process of learning and growing and changing.

It is not, however, a definitive interpretation of spiritual care. It is simply offered as a set of reflections to be shared and talked about, to be changed and made use of. I hope, therefore, that it can be another tool for those who are involved with, or who simply think about, issues of spirituality in whatever form, for themselves and in working with others.

But there is another reason why the Peanuts cartoon of the pictures in the clouds is important to me. It is because it is in picture form that it communicates what I want to say better than long and detailed explanations. It is a picture which, once clear in the mind, can be used and built upon for further explorations and discussion.

This method of communication has become an important part of the way I think and am able to understand things for myself, and of the way I try to fulfil my ministry and my chaplaincy role. If I can find a picture and, more so, if I offer that picture to people so that they can connect with it and use it as a starting point for their own explorations, I find more and more that the process of shared understanding progresses smoothly and helpfully. My son tells me I speak in metaphors. I am not unhappy with that!

There are some pictures which I have used and refined as the years have gone on. There are pictures which have been given to me by other people which I have adapted and developed. There are pictures which – in answer to fervent prayers for divine guidance, along the lines of 'Lord, give me something which will be useful here!' – have popped into my mind, and which, when offered, have seemed to be exactly what was required.

So they are my metaphors, the tools of my trade. I share them with you as I have shared them with those with whom I have worked. They may be of help to you in your own understanding of the issues you work with in your own life. But I hope, too, that through you they might be useful to other people as you seek to offer them a way of expressing themselves and understanding something of their present and future circumstances.

I have heard it said that the role of the hospice chaplain is to help people 'articulate their longings'. That has to be right. Faced with a need for living, a desire to make sense of the jumbled mess which has tumbled out of the Pandora's box, longings cry out to be articulated. One way I try to do that is with pictures like these.

I have been using some of these pictures for a very long time. Others, on the other hand, are very new and rough. But I hope that at least they will be the beginning of a process of reflection and looking at things in a different way.

What do I see in the clouds? A duckie and a horsie, sometimes. But, unlike Charlie Brown, I will bother to share my pictures with you, not to make spirituality and the practice of spiritual care simple – for it is not that! – but to offer something to the growing awareness of its importance, and to show that it can be effective.

So let me begin with a simple picture, a practical example from what I am sure lies in your own experience to know and understand. It is a picture which is as applicable to our work as carers, in whatever capacity, of those who are weak and vulnerable, as it is to an understanding of the nature of God, as people in their struggles of faith and doubt seek to discern and understand God with them on the journey. And for those who are charged with the task of telling stories to children, in church or school services, for example, here is a vivid and practical message-in-picture-form which might be of use.

Crossing a busy road, especially where there is no pelican crossing or the like, can be very dangerous. Even adults get scared sometimes, especially in busy city streets. So children should cross with a grown-up, and should hold hands tightly all the way across until they are safe on the other side.

Holding hands with someone you trust is important. But there are two ways of holding hands (and if I'm doing this in a service I'll take two children out to the front with me to act out the two different ways). The first is for the child to say, 'Please may I hold your hand!' and grip on to the grown-up's hand and start off across the road. But, you see, because it's the child who is holding on, when there are distractions and temptations, where there is a loss of concentration or if you are tired holding on with a firm grip, you may let go and part company from the safe, adult hand. You are now in danger in the middle of the road. (It's great fun to get a child to do this with you and then let go and allow them to sit down with the others when they are no longer holding your hand. Very visual!)

But there's another way of holding hands across a busy street, and that is to say, 'Please will you hold my hand?' Now the child's hand is held firmly by the big, grown-up hand, and no matter how tired, distracted or weak the child might get, the grown-up hand will hold firm and the dangerous road will be crossed safely. (This bit is even more fun with a child. Tell them to go and sit down while you are still holding on to their hand. Of course they can't, and the point – even more visually effective – is well made!)

Carers are like that, promising to hold on with their love when those in need are struggling, distracted, weak or vulnerable. And God's love? Well, it's not hard to see the connection, is it? It is not the strength of faith that matters, but the grace of God, the love that never lets go. Make use of the picture as you will.

The Roman poet Virgil wrote, 'They reached out their hands in longing for a further shore.' It is a human characteristic to want to reach out to make it through the dangers of the journey. But, in doing so, do we not so often need a safe and caring hand to hold us firm?

In religious terms, Minnie Louise Haskins, a retired lecturer at the London School of Economics, put it so well when she wrote as an introduction to her poem 'The Desert', written in 1908, the lines quoted by King George VI in a Christmas broadcast in 1939:

And I said to the man who stood at the gate of the year: 'Give me a light that I may tread safely into the unknown.' And he replied: 'Go out into the darkness and put your hand into the hand of God. That shall be to you better than light and safer than a known way.'

So, a picture – in actual or metaphorical presentation – can be more effective than mere words or explanations. And it is all about practical guidance for living in its human and its religious aspects. For which of us does not need some new insights? And which of us cannot learn something from new pictures and illustrations?

Perhaps that's why, more and more, I think and speak in pictures. Maybe it is because they are for me often better than words, more profound, more real, drawing the hearer into the picture so that they can begin and continue their own exploration, and not be trapped by my limited explanation through my limited words.

And perhaps that's why my home is filled with pictures – all speaking to me in their own way of people and places, of events and memories – telling me their stories over and over again, stories I'll never tire of hearing.

John Levering's picture

John gave me the picture before he died.
For John was an artist,
and a beautiful man,
in his heart,
by his faith,
and with his artist's hands.
And his beauty,
his love with Sarah,
his commitment to his God,
changed my life.

John gave me the picture before he died.
For he had listened to me
as I unfolded my search
for fullness of life,
for deepening of faith,
and for beauty
in me.
He had listened –
for that was his gift –
as I offered insights –
from Iona, my spiritual home,
from family,
from faith,
from my journey so far.
He had listened to me in his dying.

John gave me the picture before he died –
wild geese in flight,
painted from what he had seen
and known
and understood
of faith
and life
and the soaring of Canada geese –
wild geese in flight,
wings outstretched
for their journey.

John gave me the picture before he died.
And he had offered no words of explanation,
for none were needed.

John gave me the picture before he died.
And now I look at the picture
and see seven geese still flying,
untiring on their journey on,
and I see John,
and Sarah,
and God,
and I give thanks for their beauty
always
with me.

John gave me the picture before he died,
and I have its beauty still.

A prayer for this day

God of the dawning, grant me hope for this day
that I may walk in your pathway and live in your light.

God of the morning, grant me purpose to go forward
to respond to the promise of opportunities to love and serve.

God of the noontide, grant me strength as I labour to serve,
to keep my head high, and fulfil my commitment to the task.

God of the rest-hour, grant me grace to be still,
to know the healing balm of time alone, and to find you in the peace.

God of the evening, grant me space and time
to let go of my responsibilities,
to enjoy the pleasures of rest and the company of those I love.

God of the night, grant me the faith to face the darkness without fear,
to know that you will hold me in the blessed sleep of time and eternity.

God of all my days, grant me the promise of days yet to come,
and the thankfulness of past days well used.

Two

The traveller in the desert

And yonder all before us lie deserts of vast eternity
Andrew Marvell: To His Coy Mistress

A voice cries out, 'Prepare in the wilderness a road for the Lord!'
Isaiah 40:3

At the heart of being human is a spiritual experience which may be challenged and dislocated in the face of life-threatening illness. The value of chaplaincy, therefore, is the recognition of this dimension in order that people can be supported in their search for meaning, faith and hope, and be enabled to recognise the wholeness of life within dying and death.

These words, encapsulated in the definition of chaplaincy within Marie Curie Cancer Care, sum up my experience as a chaplain, and indeed touch on the experience of all who work in hospice care.

In the face of death people find – perhaps for the first time in their lives – that they are 'dislocated', thrown into places which are unfamiliar, with feelings that are new and strange and often very frightening. They are removed from the comfortable surroundings which have given them security and a framework for their living – home, job, salary, pension, family, purpose and even religious belief. It is not only about being a patient in a hospital or hospice where the physical surroundings are unfamiliar; it is also about what people experience within themselves, what they feel. It is an issue of the spirit as well as the body or mind. In their 'being' they are dis-located, ending up in a place which they have never inhabited before.

Ian was a man in his mid-forties, and he was struggling with the reality that he was going to die. One day he said to me: 'When I was told that there was no cure for my cancer and that all that could be offered was palliation of my symptoms but no alteration in the process of my disease, my overwhelming feeling was that somehow a chain had been broken. I felt completely disconnected from the past and with no hold of a future. I kept saying, "I have never been in this position before. What should I think? How should I feel? What should I be doing?" I felt like an alien on a strange planet where nothing made sense any more.'

What Ian was experiencing was this sense of dislocation, the link with normality being broken. All of a sudden he had been thrown into a place which was unfamiliar and strange and frightening.

I recognise this feeling often in my work with dying and bereaved people. In different guises it comes up over and over again. And so it has created the first of my pictures in my understanding of spiritual care – that of a lost traveller in a desert, a picture I hold regularly in my mind when I work with people like Ian to help me understand what they feel and experience, and to keep hold of the purpose of my being with them in the first place.

If this 'dislocation' concept is as real as I believe it to be, then dying people are often in a wilderness where there are no signposts to guide them across a barren and frightening wasteland to another place of security, or even back to the familiar, safe place from which they have come. Often there are not even any paths for them to walk, far less signposts – no well trodden routes others have marked out by their journeys before them. For as far as they can see, there is barren, trackless waste with no horizon, no way of knowing which way to go, or whether the desert will ever have an end.

Is it any wonder, therefore, that people in this desert place, this place of dislocation, are fearful in the face of death? It is not the fact of death which induces that fear. From the moment of birth, or should we say from the dawn of understanding of the nature of our living, we know – in our heads, at least – that life is finite and that one day all shall die. It is the process of the journey to death which is frightening, being on that journey with no familiar landmarks, or sense of direction, or purpose, or clarity, or hope... It is the realisation that we are in that desert alone, with no sense of companionship, and in religious terms – echoing the devastation of the Psalmist – even feeling abandoned by God.

In light of this image of the lost traveller in the desert, it is the task of the carer, in the general sense of our caring for the sick and dying, and in the specific sense of offering spiritual care, to enter into that place of dislocation and express a commitment to be with that person in their desert wanderings. If the loneliness and fear felt by someone in the face of death is to be understood and taken seriously, then the carer has to begin by recognising the sense of dislocation of the dying person by being the fellow traveller who will help to dispel the fear of being alone. Our primary task is to go to that lost traveller in the desert so that they are no longer alone in their frightening wilderness.

We have to take the time simply to be there for each patient or person we work with – as Metropolitan Anthony Bloom writes: '... not just sitting looking vaguely and vacantly about ... but going deep, so deep in sympathy, in compassion that your presence speaks, and if there is need, you can put your hand on the person and it will mean more than whatever you can say.'

To go to the lost traveller, to offer them your presence, to be in that 'deep' place with them, offers compassion and healing more powerfully than I had ever realised before.

I cannot alter the fact that someone is going to die. I cannot give them the one thing they want above all else, to be told that it is all a bad dream, that there is a miracle cure, that death has been cheated. I have said often enough to patients and carers that I wished I could wave a magic wand and make all this pain and sorrow go away, but I can't. So am I to do what the dying person has seen others do – to turn my back in my uselessness and walk away, abandoning that person to their ultimate fate?

Or am I to go to them in their loneliness and share their pain? To acknowledge the fact of your impotence to change the reality of death is to admit to that patient or carer that you are already standing where they stand, that in your being you are with them. If the environment for dying people is the desert, then that is where the caring relationship must start, and that is where hope begins to be renewed.

However, for me as a chaplain, the image needs to be taken a little further. I have my own personal system of beliefs, my purpose for living or whatever you would call it, which gives me my own security and peace of mind. It is as if I have found a settlement surrounded by a strong wall that gives me a protective security against the ravages of the desert outside. (At least, in my best moments that is how I feel! The description of that settlement, the nature of its walls, the layout of its streets, the height of its battlements need not be detailed here, for that place for me has been developed, changed and redefined over many years and through many circumstances. Such is the nature of faith.)

As I look out over the desert wastes from the security of my settlement, sometimes I become aware of a lost traveller, because I hear their distant cry or see their predicament from afar. If I then simply stay in my place of safety and call out instructions, I do nothing to help. I take no risk when I play safe and choose to remain distant and separate.

If, on the other hand, I do decide to launch forth on a rescue mission but do so with a pre-prepared plan or a map to guide the dislocated person to safety, the motives for my caring are questionable and the outcome of my intervention problematic. For there are no ready answers or pat solutions which will rescue the desert traveller and whisk them off to safety as if by magic. The outcome of the journey together may be a sense of purpose or direction, or even some answers to big questions. But it is not, and should not be, the initial purpose. And to meet the traveller with a solution already worked out is to offer them *my* journey and not to help them to find their own.

I believe it is vital that carers have their own place of security and strength from which to launch into the desert and to return to for their own strengthening and inner renewal. (I'll say a little more about this in a later chapter using another picture of houses and attics.) It is scary going into the desert to experience some of the 'lostness' of the forlorn traveller. We need a place of safety to which we can return. But it is taking the risk of abandoning our security and entering into the desert for a while that makes spiritual care a reality. So, in order to accompany the lost and dislocated traveller, there has to be a commitment to listen and not to offer instant solutions; to hear the cries of anguish and not to judge or condemn; and to be aware of the struggle for direction and purpose, and to wait with patience until it is time to move on.

I recall Sam and his family. Sam was in a single room in our Centre and, while I knew him a little, I had never met his wife and two children, as they always seemed to have been around when I wasn't. Sam had taken a turn for the worse, and his wife, son and daughter had been called in during the night. When I came in the following morning, they were sitting quietly by Sam's bed. His wife had red eyes. His daughter was sobbing. His son was staring blankly out of the window. They were dignified and caring, but obviously distraught. I knew all of this because I could see them through the open door of the room as I walked by. And having seen the distress, I did the only thing I felt I could do – I went to our coffee-room for a cup of tea!

I did not want to enter that room, so I walked right past it many times that morning. I was simply frightened to go in because I had nothing to say. I rationalised it by telling myself I did not want to intrude on the privacy of a family or that I had other pressing things to do. In actual fact, I ducked it because I felt so useless. I had nothing to offer. The nurses were superb. They couldn't duck it. They were in and out, doing what they do extraordinarily well. But it wasn't for me.

Eventually I realised this could not go on. There was that little voice in my head asking me how I could live with myself if I did nothing. So, later in the day, I took a big deep breath and in I went. I said hello. I put a hand on a shoulder. I said I wished I could say something really clever, but I wasn't going to try. But I assured them we were around when we were needed. I was there for five minutes or so. I did that a few times that day. Each time I felt awkward. I felt I had achieved nothing, only the satisfaction that I could go home knowing that I had not ducked it altogether.

Sam died that night. The following morning when the family returned to collect the death certificate and Sam's belongings, his wife asked to see me. She asked me to conduct Sam's funeral service. I agreed to do so, and we arranged to meet the following day to go over the details. As she was leaving, she held my hand and said thank you for my support – and specifically for my help the previous day. I mumbled something about not giving very much. And she said, 'But you did. You came into our room, and I know how hard that must have been for you.'

I was floored! But, you see, whatever had happened, a family had known that the chaplain, with all his inadequacy and fearfulness, had met them in the desert of that single room, and they took more peace and comfort from that than I could ever have realised. They genuinely felt that along with all their practical needs their spiritual needs had been cared for too – simply because the threshold had been crossed.

One dictionary defines hospice as 'a place of rest for travellers'. But before the weary traveller finds that place of rest on the journey, they have a need to be met in the desert so that they do not have to face their fearful journey alone.

Duncan was Sam's son. After his father died he showed me a poem he'd written which he asked me to read at the funeral, because he wanted to express something of how he felt about the people who had cared for his father, himself and his family, and how he hoped people would continue to come to them in their need. With his permission I share it with you.

If you've never stood in that man's shoes
or saw things through his eyes,
or stood and watched with helpless hands
while the heart inside you dies …
So help each other along the way
no matter where you start;
for the same God that made him, made us too,
these souls with broken hearts.

I don't expect anyone can really stand in another person's shoes to experience all that they experience and feel all that they feel. But unless we seek to express our empathy, and at least try to come close – and, sometimes, watch with helpless hands too – can we truly say that we have even begun to understand?

The Canadian singer/songwriter James Keelaghan writes this in one of his songs:

Take a walk under my skies;
Try to see things once the way I do;
Take a look out through my eyes;
Take a different point of view.
Everything changes,

Every fact wears some disguise.
Cast off your troubles —
Take a walk under my skies.

Sometimes that walk will be scary. Sometimes looking through someone else's eyes will mean you will despair as they despair, and cry as they cry. But there is no doubt that it works, and as you meet them in their place of dislocation the loneliness of the journey of suffering and dying is, at least for a moment, accepted and understood.

The meeting place

No one told me it was going to be like this.
'Carry on with the pathway,' they said,
'Just follow the signs.
You'll be OK.
That's what it's all about.
Have faith.
Keep going.
Carry on!'

What pathway?
It's been worn away by the winds and desert storms.
Someone might have been along this way only yesterday.
But you'd never know.
And what signs?
Where are they now?
Did I miss them?
Were they never here at all?
Was it all a con?

No one told me it was going to be like this.

*

People said it would be like this.
Pretty good, eh?
Sheltered in the city,
big, strong walls,
guards on the gate,
lookouts on the ramparts,

and good people around.
Yes, it's as good as they said,
and, boy, am I glad this city is here.

People said it would be like this.
Thank God we can keep the desert at bay,
making sure the unrelenting wilderness,
with its fear and its danger
is kept firmly in its place.

Yes, indeed, it's really good to be here.

People said it would be like this.

                    *

No one told me it would be like this,
no hope …
no hope …
no …
But … there … there …
It can't be …
Is it real?
Good God!
There's a city wall,
there, in the distance.
No, I'm not going mad,
it's there, right enough.
Help!

Is anyone there?
Oh, I'm too tired to get there,
too weary to shout loud enough.

No one told me it would be like this.
A city ...
out of reach?
It might as well be miles away,
out of sight ...
No chance ...
of ...
shelter ...

No one told me it would be like this.

*

People said it would be like this.
I can stand here,
high up on my city wall
and know that I'm always safe.
I can look out and see the desert
and know it's no danger to me.
I can look out and see ...
and see ...
Good God!
There's someone out there.
There!
In the desert!

No one told me it would be like this.
There …
Someone …
Who?
Why?
And what do I do?
Is no one else going to do anything?
Do I have to go,
out there,
into that?

No one told me it would be like this.

*

No one told me it would be like this.
To die alone,
when all that was promised was a clear pathway,
a well-trodden journey from there to there.
But here,
now,
it's all hopeless,
and the city might as well not be there.

No one told me it would be like this.
And the city …
that city …
that city …

Good God, that city …
What?
Is it real?
Someone's coming …
Yes …
From the city …
Someone's decided to come …
It's going to be OK!

People said it would be like this.

*

'People said it would be like this, my friend.
People said it would be like this.
And they were right.
God be with you on your travels.
Safe journey.
Go well.'

'And you, my friend.
And all the best to the people of your city.
Go well.'

Good God,
people said it would be like this.
People said …
and they were right.

A prayer of thanks for healing love

She came, Lord, to my bedside,
a nurse of tender years,
younger than my granddaughter,
a mere slip of a girl.
She came, Lord, to me,
aged and frail,
sick and weak,
and I doubted what she could do for me.
She touched, Lord, with tender hands
my wrinkled skin and bony frame,
with gentle skill
and knowing look.
She touched, Lord, my life with love –
beyond my weakened body,
she reached my very soul.
She healed, Lord, my broken life,
my furrowed brow,
my wasted muscles tensed with pain,
my sullen look,
my very face turned away from any gaze.
She healed, Lord, and gave me time
to learn again to take and not reject such tender love.
She healed, Lord,
and gave me hope.

She loved, Lord,
she loved even me,
the me of such frailty and brokenness
such dying and hopelessness
that I doubted whether anyone could love,
whether I could love, whether You could love.
She came, Lord, and she loved me as I am.
She came, and touched, and healed, and loved,
and went away
that others, too, might know.

Three

The companion on the journey

I have had playmates, I have had companions,
In my days of childhood, my joyful school days —
All, all are gone, the old familiar faces.
Charles Lamb: The Old Familiar Faces

In the dark days we need the refuge of friendship.
Jean Vanier: Community and Growth

All of us who work in health care need to remember that we are people first and professionals second. Often it is the people part of us that is required most in our offering of spiritual care.

Spirituality is integral to life, and every life is unique. There is, therefore, a need to recognise the uniqueness of each individual in order to provide a caring and loving environment where patients can feel at ease.

In medieval times, hospices were nothing to do with the care of dying people. Instead, they were places of hospitality, usually attached to monasteries and run by monastic orders. They were places of rest and renewal for the travellers on the pilgrim routes through Europe, staging-posts for holy pilgrims on their journey of faith and commitment. So the modern hospice movement has as its focus the creation of a 'place of rest for travellers', but now they are travellers on the journey of life, for whom the journey has been a hard one, and whose onward journey may well be problematic.

As the body needs nourishment for the journey, so too does the soul, and as carers in the hospice setting we are in the position to provide this nourishment. To do so we have to listen and to help people tell the story of who they are, to express their own fears and uncertainties, to share their own joys and sorrows.

This has always been fundamental. The need to focus on the patient – for hospice care to be 'patient centred' or 'patient led' – is a key to what we do and what we stand for.

In the field of spiritual care this is even more important. Indeed, it is perhaps all the more crucial in this facet of care to go with the person with whom we are working, because there will have been others – perhaps even in the intimacy of the family circle – who have either abandoned the loved one to their fears and anxieties because they cannot handle what is coming up, or who have jumped quickly to facile judgements and condemnation, or offered simplistic solutions. It is easy to stop listening. It is easy to listen and condemn. It is easy to trot out platitudes. In all these responses what the patient experiences is rejection, and a further deepening of their sense of being alone in their struggles.

I remember Frank being admitted to our Centre late one afternoon. He was a man in his mid-sixties, and he was very frail and only semi-conscious. He had been cared for at home until it was too much for those who were looking after him. When he was admitted, he was accompanied by a woman and a man of similar age to himself. The woman was his wife. And the man was his best friend. While Frank was being examined by a doctor, his two companions were also cared for and given a reassuring cup of tea. I happened to be around and was introduced to them as well, offering further gentle reassurance and comfort. As I was leaving them, the gentleman took me aside and asked for a private word. 'I want to explain our relationship to someone,' he said. So, in a private corner, he did just that. 'Frank,' he said, 'is bisexual. The three of us have lived as a *menage à trois* for 18 years. He has relations with both of us – separately, you understand.' I nodded sagely, as if I was told this kind of thing every day of the week! And the man concluded, 'I needed to tell someone so that you would be aware of the depth of our relationships together.'

Frank died that night. The next morning I was asked to go and see the couple at their request. Once again I was invited by them to conduct the funeral service. And while I was exploring things with them, it became clear to me that what I was dealing with was two grieving partners, both experiencing the loss of their lover and friend. I knew a voice was screaming inside me, 'I don't understand this! I can't really make any sense of it! What am I going to say? Get me out of here!'

Just at that point I was asked, 'Will you have to say we are forgiven for the way we have lived? Will you have to mention it in the service?' I replied: 'You do not need to be forgiven, in private or in public, for you have done nothing wrong. You will not be judged or condemned.'

I may not have understood. And the lifestyle of these three people was certainly not mine. But it was not my place, then or now, to judge or condemn. It was my role to listen, to journey with those people in their need, their loss and their grief. It was my ministry to offer the Grace of God. If there had been the smallest flicker of judgement, any moment of healing would have been lost, and God would have been perceived as unloving.

I am convinced that there is in our Scottish psyche the brooding presence of a dour, black-cloaked Presbyterian minister who is constantly wagging his finger at us and condemning us as sinners! Can there be any other reason why these grieving people had to seek reassurance that the Church would not point a finger of blame at them for their lifestyle when what they needed was compassion and comfort?

And in case the Presbyterians think they have cornered the market in self-criticism, Rabbi Harold Kushner affirms that in the human psyche there is an infinite capacity for guilt. So if people are hearing voices of condemnation, of judgement, of banishment –

from the Church as well as elsewhere – it only serves to reinforce the capacity for guilt which is already inherent in their human nature. How dare we add to that and continually reinforce the burden and sense of rejection people feel! Instead, let us enter into their world, listen to their story, track with their feelings and fears – and show them the love and mercy of God in action.

A person's journey may not be our way. They may not respond to a set of circumstances as we ourselves would. But it is their inherent freedom to choose their attitude, to choose their own way. Is it not, therefore, our responsibility to enhance that freedom, to seek to understand the way they have chosen to travel, and to journey with them on their road?

The picture which helps me understand this role in spiritual care comes from the writings of Dr Sheila Cassidy. Her book, *Sharing the Darkness*, written in the context of her work as Medical Director of St Luke's Hospice, Plymouth, was a formative influence on me in my early years in hospice chaplaincy.

I can do no better than allow Dr Cassidy to speak for herself:

The dying ... are essentially people on a journey. They are uprooted people, dispossessed, marginalised, travelling fearfully into the unknown ... Sometimes the movement is barely perceptible, like the moving floors at Heathrow, but sometimes the tracks hurtle through the night, throwing their bewildered occupants from side to side with all the terror of the line to Auschwitz. Above all, the dying are alone and they are afraid. So the spirituality of those who care for the dying must be the spirituality of the companion, of the friend who walks alongside, helping, sharing, and sometimes just sitting, empty-handed, when he would rather run away. It is the spirituality of presence, of being alongside, watchful, available, of being there.

The picture, therefore, is one of the companion on the journey. It is what has been described as 'incarnational theology', believing that your presence with an individual in their need is enough. How hard it is to put into practice! How often have I felt that I needed to say something or do something when what was required was simply to be there and let healing take place.

In any hospice, it is not surprising that families and friends of patients come back days or weeks after their loved one has died to say thank you to the staff. Our hospice is no different. There are always 'thank you' cards on the notice-board to be shared with all the staff, and there always seem to be boxes of chocolates available in the Duty Rooms given to us by grateful people.

Often the opportunity to return to the place where the death has occurred is an important hurdle to get over in the grieving process. And we as staff need to make contact with people again too, to see how they are getting on and to continue to express our care.

One day a lady arrived on the wards whom I recognised, but whose name, to be honest, I could not recall. I could not even remember the patient whom she had been visiting. In any event, she spent time with the nursing team in the Duty Room, gave them a box of chocolates as a thank you, and took her leave. I met her in the corridor. She greeted me warmly and I did likewise – still struggling to remember who she was! She thanked me for my help for her and her husband – at least I knew now that it was her husband we had had as a patient! – and I muttered something in response. 'No,' she continued, 'I want to say thank you specifically for your help the day my husband died, when I came in to see him, and you met me at the front door. Without that I don't think I would have been able to face that day and the days that followed. So thank you.'

Now, the front door of our Centre lies between the reception area and the toilet, or on the way to the Day Centre. I have absolutely no recollection of the meeting to which this lady referred. Almost certainly I would have been on my way to the loo or the Day Centre, and would have bumped into her as she arrived. But whatever happened, the moment of meeting was a moment of companionship, of eye contact, of focus, of touch, of reassurance, of love. And so it was a moment of healing and of strength, not of my doing, but of a greater purpose than mine and facilitated by that chance meeting. It was an encounter that she could take with her as a contribution to her needs when the actual interaction was over. It was, therefore, a moment of spiritual care.

Another quite different incident had essentially the same outcome. It was a series of short but regular meetings with Sally whose mother was a patient, close to death. Our relationship was not extraordinary of itself or unique in its content. But it was built on times of companionship. In fact, I spent most of my time with Sally sitting on the floor beside her and her mother's bed. We were relaxed together, talking, sharing, and sometimes laughing too. On one occasion Sally said: 'I feel I am on a hectic journey, on a bus travelling too fast, with no clear destination, on a road I have never seen before, with no landmarks and familiar sights. It's a rough ride, and made all the worse because I am on the bus alone.' My task, and the task of all who cared for her in any way during the journey of her mother's death and through bereavement, was to get on the bus with her, to experience the rough ride, to stay on the bus still it stopped, to reassure, to comfort, or simply to be there. It is the companion role again, sharing the fear and the darkness. And I have no doubt that it works.

The companion of the dying person, therefore, or indeed of anyone who is experiencing the 'dark night of the soul', has to be prepared to enter into their darkness, to journey with them along their strange and scary road. As Sheila Cassidy writes:

This is the meaning of compassion: to enter into the suffering of another, to share in some small way in their pain, confusion and desolation.

I would add also that it is a privilege to be that person who is trusted enough to be invited to share the journey. To be a companion to dying people is never easy, but it is enormously rewarding.

I have often heard nurses and other health care professionals who have begun to grasp the importance of spiritual care say: 'I don't know what to do. I have nothing to say. I feel I have nothing to offer. Give us the tools and equip us for the job.' To which I respond that there is no guidebook, no manual of spiritual care. But to walk away in our uselessness is to duck it, and is to deny the patient or struggling family member the worth of our presence.

As I have already indicated, every person has spiritual needs. But often these needs have been neglected, by theorists, teachers and practitioners alike. The reason for this omission may be because spirituality cannot be easily quantified. But I suspect that it is also because we as carers are ill at ease with our own spirituality, and not able, therefore, to appreciate fully the spiritual needs of the people for whom we care.

It is not surprising, therefore, that there are no procedures, 'nothing we can say'. But to duck the issue altogether is to deny the person who is fearful on the journey to death the healing power which comes from our being with them, a companion on the journey, when so many others in their embarrassment and inadequacy have abandoned them to their fate.

I conclude this chapter with the words of a song by John L. Bell. I have read these words at funeral services when I have been very much aware of the brokenness of people's lives, the inadequacies of our living which are all too obvious, and the many questions which remain about failure and suffering and death – and when I have been devastatingly aware that, above all, I have nothing to say.

I do not believe it is our task to answer the questions people throw at us, but to be that living presence which the incarnation of Christ embodies. It is our task to affirm in our 'being' with people on their journey the validity of their pain and their questions, and to point to the living, 'companioning' presence of God.

All the fears I need not name but am too scared to say:
all the shame for what I've done which nothing can allay;
all the people I've let down and lost along the way:
all the hate I still remand.
    Must these torment me to the end of time?
    Who is there to understand?

All the wasted years in which I've struggled to be free;
all the broken promises that took their toll on me;
all the love I should have shown and all I failed to be;
all I longed to take my hand.
    Must these torment me to the end of time?
    Who is there to understand?

What the cause of pain is and, much more, the reason why;
what my final hour will bring, how suddenly I'll die;
what the future holds for those I'll miss, for whom I cry;
what, too late, I might demand.
    Shall these torment me to the end of time?
    Who is there to understand?

'All the wrong you now admit, I promise to forgive;
all that you regret you are not sentenced to relive;
all the love you've never known is mine alone to give;
you, my child, are understood.
    So do not fear all that is yet to be:
    heaven is close and God is good.'

The journey

It wasn't the journey which made me afraid.
It was being alone.
Oh, I know I was scared when I came aboard.
Why was I here?
Where was I going?
How long would it take?
What would the journey be like?
You bet, I was scared,
fearful of the unknown,
of how I'd cope,
of what the outcome would be.
And I sat there,
very frightened indeed.

And then I looked around,
and I realised I was alone.
Where were all the rest,
the ones I'd been with only a moment ago?
Where were all the ones who said they would come too,
who'd never leave me
or forsake me
or abandon me to my fate?
Where were they when I needed them most?
I was overwhelmed with panic.
You have to face the journey, they said.

But they never said it would be like this.
They never told me how it would feel.
And who was there to tell?
Who would know?
Who would care?

God, I'm frightened.
I don't know what's happening to me.
I don't know what will happen next.
I don't know what it will be like.
And I'm alone – alone – ALONE.

I don't remember when she came aboard.
Maybe she'd been there for ages, and I hadn't noticed,
or maybe she'd just come on.
But there she was,
just a few seats away,
nearer the front,
sitting quietly,
reading a magazine.

She didn't look like someone I knew.
A stranger, then.
But better an unknown stranger who was there
than a friend who'd promised to come and hadn't bothered!
I wanted to shout hello
or run towards her down the aisle,
and sit beside her
and touch her just to prove she was real.
But I didn't.
Well, you don't, do you?
I just sat and looked at her for ages.

And once,
just once,
she turned around,
and smiled.

And I looked out of the window
as the journey began.
And as we travelled,
I saw things I knew
and I saw things I didn't recognise at all.
And sometimes the journey was very slow
and sometimes it was fast and bumpy
and very scary.

But not frightening.
No, not frightening.
Just scary sometimes,
but not mind-numbing, overwhelming frightening again,
not ever again.

And the stranger never moved.
She just stayed,
there,
sharing the journey.
And sometimes
she would turn
and smile.

A prayer for strength

Give me the strength, Lord, to take another step, when all seems lost,
and I'm too weary now to move again.

Give me the patience, Lord, when progress still is slow,
and future steps seem far too hard to contemplate.

Give me the courage, Lord, when twists and turns
obscure the open way and make me sore afraid.

Give me the wisdom, Lord, to trust your promise made to me,
that if you've been with me in days gone by
you will not leave my side when times are hard.

Give me the faith then, Lord, that when I do not know that you are there
I might believe that in the mystery you stay.

Give me the purpose, Lord, that when a weary traveller comes my way,
to know in that companionship you are my guide and strength and stay.

Give me the hope, Lord, I now need to onward go
and know the journey will not be in vain.

Four

Sharing the tears

If you have tears, prepare to shed them now.
William Shakespeare: Julius Caesar

Laugh and the world laughs with you, weep and you weep alone.
Ella Wheeler Wilcox: Solitude

The question 'Why?' is common in the face of death. It is expressed in many ways: 'Why am I being punished when people worse than me are fine?' 'Why does God allow this to happen?' 'Why my daughter?' 'Why suffering?' 'Why now?' 'Why me?' These questions create anxieties in all of us, regardless of whether we are involved with hospice care or not, simply because we are human.

As carers it is as if we are cast in the role of parent who is expected to be the fountain of all knowledge, to whom the vulnerable child comes with questions and the need for answers. Not surprisingly, therefore, the question 'Why?' is commonplace. And not surprisingly it creates anxieties when it is raised, in whatever form it comes up.

I recall an occasion when I was a child going to an ice-rink with my mother, father and sister. My sister and I sat with my dad watching my mother skating around – or at least we watched while my dad, as usual, had his nose buried in his daily paper. I was an inquisitive child, so I asked what for me was the obvious question: 'Dad, how do you get ice on an ice-rink when it isn't frosty outside?' After all, wasn't my father the fountain of all knowledge? Isn't that what dads are for? Without a moment's hesitation – and without lifting his head from his paper – my father replied: 'It's all done by means of an electric plant, son.' Fine! I had no problem with that. An electric plant. Sounded good to me!

I know now what my father meant then. But, for more years than I care to remember, I had a picture in my head of how they get ice on an ice-rink – a green, tendrilly thing under the ice, all cold and frosty, making the ice for the ice-rink, and plugged in somewhere – at least I understood the electric bit! I trusted my father's knowledge. I believed what he told me.

My father, I suppose, felt he should offer something by way of an answer, maybe to shut this child up so he could concentrate on his paper, or maybe simply to be dismissive of an inquisitive little boy. But I suspect it was also something about not wanting to lose face, not wanting to fail in his role. (My son told me once that he could never remember me saying 'I don't know' in answer to one of his probing questions. Like father, like son!)

As carers, we are given – or are happy to take on – the mantle of the all-knowing parent to the questioning child. And we become so familiar with that role that we try to give answers even when we do not have any or, indeed, when there are none! How often, therefore, have we felt that knot in the stomach that wouldn't go away because we felt we had failed. We didn't have a ready answer. There was no procedure to be implemented, no form of words to fit appropriately and relieve the questioner's anxiety, fear or distress. So we are racked with our own questions and sense of failure: 'What do I say?' 'What do I do?' 'What do I have to offer at moments like these?'

Chaplains are not immune to the stress of these moments either. But I have found that there are a few basic principles which can help. For one thing – as I have already indicated – there is no rule book, no standard, no manual of procedures that will equip you with the right things to say. It just isn't possible.

But it is looking at the whole issue from another angle that has created for me another picture which I have found helpful. The question 'Why?', and other questions in the face of death, are not questions, they are cries of pain. Viewed in this way, they do not need answers. But they do need comfort.

The image which arises from this comes to me from Rabbi Harold Kushner, author of a very helpful book, *When Bad Things Happen to Good People*. He tells the story of a little boy whose mother sends him on an errand and it takes him a long time to get back. When he finally returns, his worried mother says to him, 'Where were you? I was fearful for you.' And the boy says, 'There's a kid down the street whose tricycle broke and he was crying 'cause he couldn't fix it. And I felt sorry for him so I stopped to help him.' His mother says, 'Are you trying to tell me you know how to fix a tricycle?' The kid says, 'No, of course not. But I sat down and helped him cry.'

The picture, therefore, is one of sharing the tears. People who utter the cries of pain contained within the question 'Why?' do not need them rationalised away with a clever response. They need to have them accepted for what they are: cries of devastation and helplessness. Kushner affirms:

When you cannot fix what is broken, you can help very profoundly by sitting down and helping someone cry. A person who is suffering does not want explanation: the person wants consolation. Not reasons, but reassurance.

Take the image closer to home, again from the parent/child perspective. When a child in your care falls and grazes a knee and comes to you with screams of anguish, do you give them a detailed treatise on the meaning of suffering, or a physiological explanation of the nature of pain? I think not. Instead, you take the child onto your knee and hold them, hug them until the tears and sobs subside. They need a physical – or metaphorical – hug of comfort.

So patients and families need to be listened to in like fashion. They need to be affirmed where they are. They need to have their cries accepted as valid, and not explained away. They need to be embraced – tears and all.

Emerging spiritual needs are often revealed in painful questions. As these questions tumble out from the Pandora's box, they come from the depth of a person's being; they are what I have heard described as 'stirrings of the soul'. Answers to such questions are unknown and unknowable. But hearing them, accepting them, and being responsive to them means that we are in the realm of the spirit, deeply involved with spiritual issues, and beginning to meet the needs expressed.

It is not failure on our part to have no answers to the questions. It is exactly the opposite. To accept the questions as cries and, on occasions, to share tears with the broken and anguished person, is to participate in profound moments of spiritual healing.

Caring for those we cannot cure, being with those who constantly ask 'Why?', listening to a depth of feeling with all its pain is hard, especially when we are anxious about what to say in response. So, if you have nothing to say, say nothing! You have already done a great deal by affirming someone where they are and listening to their story.

What people need most is for others to 'hang in there' in their anguish and suffering. I am convinced that those who ask these questions know there are no answers. But they have seen people who can't handle the anxiety this creates simply leave them in their confusion. Healing takes place by staying with it while others run away.

No words, no platitudes, no biblical quotation can take the pain away. But the fact is people already know that there is nothing you can say. It is already part of our common humanity. And they have seen others turn away, embarrassed by their uselessness. Anyone who moves towards that broken person, and is not repulsed by their cries or their own sense of inadequacy – who, as I have said, is prepared to step over the threshold of the place they inhabit – gives confidence that they do have something to offer at moments of utter despair and reassurance that all is not lost.

It is not the voice which says: 'Don't just stand there, do something' which needs to be heeded. It is the voice which says: 'Don't do something, don't even say anything, just stand there, sit there, be there, in their need.' And it works.

I was reflecting on this with a hospice chaplain colleague a little while ago, and he told me a story from his own work. It was about a patient in his hospice, a man who had had a tracheotomy following surgery for cancer of the throat, and with whom communication by speech was very difficult. My friend would sit with him, play endless games of chess, talk too much, struggle for points of contact, and feel frustrated himself. Yet, through it all, he had been able to establish a good and trusting relationship. One day he asked the patient if he would like to come for a walk in the gardens. It was a way of sharing some time without having to speak. So, for a while, they strolled slowly in the hospice grounds, stopping occasionally to look at flowers, to point out the birds, to appreciate the warmth of the sun. Eventually, they sat down together in the shade, and stayed in silence for a long time. After a while my chaplain friend felt compelled to share something of help. So he turned to the patient and found himself saying: 'It's a bugger, isn't it?' The patient smiled, and nodded. What had needed to be said had been said. What had needed to be acknowledged had been done. And after another period of silence, chaplain and patient rose from the seat and continued their walk round the garden.

It was, my colleague reflected, one of the rare occasions when he felt he had got it absolutely right, and when he had given to a patient exactly what was needed at that time.

So we need to learn to 'be' as well as to 'do' – or at least to find a blend of both that indicates we are seeking to be truly holistic in our care. We need to value relationships and the indefinable, immeasurable qualities of caring, as well as the more quantitative aspects of care.

To value the relationship, to see being as valid as doing – and, from time to time, to recognise that we are too small or ill-equipped to fulfil the role of the fixer of the broken bike but simply to sit down and share the tears and acknowledge the pain and frustration – is to offer deep and sensitive spiritual care.

For me, this is also a profound theological issue. Have we made God too small, too quantifiable, with our knowledge of what to say and do on his behalf? Is God not bigger than our concepts, always remaining mysterious in his being? So, therefore, is it not possible that in our silence and sharing the tears, in our 'smallness' of not being fixers of everything, we are, in fact, not failing at all, but leaving room for the greatness of God to work?

I conclude this chapter, therefore, with a final story. It comes from the writings of John Taylor when he was General Secretary of the Church Missionary Society as he reflected on a theology of the Holy Spirit in a book called *The Go-between God*. It is a story which over the years has had a profound influence on me, and one which I use often in my teaching and exploration of the meaning – and the effectiveness – of spiritual care. Whether you are religious or not, it is a story which will, I hope, speak powerfully to you. I usually read it without explanation or comment. I offer it likewise here.

A colleague of mine has recently described to me an occasion when a West Indian woman in a London flat was told of her husband's death in a street accident. The shock of grief stunned her like a blow, she sank into a corner of the sofa and sat there rigid and unhearing. For a long time her terrible tranced look continued to embarrass the family, friends and officials who came and went. Then the schoolteacher of one of her children, an Englishwoman, called and, seeing how things were, went and sat beside her. Without a word she threw an arm around the tight shoulders, clasping them with her full strength. The white cheek was thrust hard against the brown. Then as the unrelenting pain seeped through to her the newcomer's tears began to flow, falling on their two hands linked in the woman's lap. For a long time that is all that was happening. And then at last the West Indian woman started to sob. Still not a word was spoken and after a little while the visitor got up and went, leaving her contribution to help the family meet its immediate needs.

That is the embrace of God, his kiss of life. That is the embrace of his mission, and of our intercession. And the Holy Spirit is the force in the straining muscles of an arm, the film of sweat between pressed cheeks, the mingled wetness on the backs of clasped hands. He is as close and as unobtrusive as that, and as irresistibly strong.

I cried

I cried with her tonight
and felt I'd let her down.
I cried when her pain touched me,
and I could not hold the tears at bay.
I cried when I felt lost with her,
and I did not know how to stop.
I did not want to cry.
I wanted to be strong,
supportive,
helpful.
But I cried with her tonight,
and I felt I'd let her down.

I did not know what to say to her tonight
and I felt I'd let myself down.
I knew I should offer some word of comfort,
some helpful consolation
from which she could have drawn strength,
something that would have made it better.
But I got all tongue-tied,
and no words came.
Tears got in the way,
and the silence was filled with her sobs and mine.
I wanted to say the right thing.
But I did not know what to say tonight
and I felt I'd let myself down.

I did not feel too Christian tonight
and I felt I'd let God down.

Yes, I went where I was needed,
called to heal and serve,
willing to cross over the road,
to love and care.
But I felt too awkward,
too ill at ease to feel I was getting it right.
Shouldn't being a Christian make it easier to care?
Why did I feel so useless?
What went wrong?
I did not feel too Christian tonight,
and I felt I'd let God down.

     *

Dear Joyce

Thank you so much for coming to see me tonight. I know it wasn't easy for you, because you've had your own struggles to face recently. But you came – and so many others haven't bothered. Thanks for the hug, and the tears. I needed to cry with you, and I'm so glad you weren't stiff and awkward like some have been. And thanks for saying nothing, and allowing the silence to help. I don't need words. I've heard platitudes till I could scream. I just needed to be held by someone who understood, and to feel safe again. I wish there were more like you, people who were human and who didn't try too hard. I really felt God was with us when you were here.

Thank you for all you've done to help me when I needed it most. I hope I can be as understanding and do the same for you some day.

With much love.
Edith

God of the moment

In the laughter you spoke to me, God,
of life and hope, of fun and purpose.
God of the laughter, I laugh with you.

In the anger you spoke to me, God,
of waste and destruction, of illness and death.
God of the anger, I am angry with you.

In the silence you spoke to me, God,
of wordless peace, of depth and calm.
God of the silence, I am silent with you.

In the comfort you spoke to me, God,
of touch and breath, of warmth and tender care.
God of the comfort, I know comfort with you.

In the tears you spoke to me, God,
of sorrow and loss, of cleansing and healing.
God of the tears, I am crying with you.

In the moment you spoke to me, God,
that moment of mystery, of wonder and love.
God of the moment, I share this moment with you.

Five

A pilot in home waters

O Captain! my Captain! our fearful trip is done,
The ship has weather'd every rack, the prize we sought is won.
Walt Whitman: O Captain! My Captain!

Sleep after toil, port after stormy seas,
Ease after war, death after life does greatly please.
Edmund Spenser: The Faerie Queen

The balance between the offer of professional care in a hospice setting and the desire to stay in the security and familiarity of one's own home is always a delicate one. Much has been done in recent years to give people options as to where their ongoing care might be carried out and, ultimately, where they would choose to die. There are times, of course, when particular facets of care and attention have to function in a specialised setting. In specific phases of the disease process, when, for example, the important issue is palliation of symptoms rather than seeking a curative process, then time in a specialist palliative care unit is an important option. But even at this stage people need the right to choose. When there are fewer and fewer choices left open to them, it has to be right that, furnished with proper information, and assured of the input of the appropriate resources, they are able to choose to stay in the familiarity of their own home if that is their overwhelming desire.

I confess that I know next to nothing of New Testament Greek. However, I do know this much about the field of medicine in which I work – the word 'palliative' has its root in the Greek word meaning to cover or shelter. So palliation of the symptoms of disease provides for people a cover or shelter from the distress they experience in the face of a life-threatening illness and the physical and emotional manifestations of its process. This means that instead of being told, 'There is nothing we can do,' because there is no cure, no procedure which will arrest the progress of the disease, people can feel and know that there is a lot that can be done. This is the gift which palliative medicine offers at moments of deep despair and hopelessness. There is a lot of positive input available which can alleviate the suffering of body, mind and spirit, and provide the best possible quality of life. The hospice setting, with its specialist palliative expertise, can provide the necessary shelter, the 'place of rest for travellers', which patients require. 'Faced with a need for living' they can be helped to 'live till they die' to the fullest extent possible.

There is still, however, a perception problem. For there is a widespread general view that hospice and palliative care is only about the terminal stage of an illness – hospices are places you go to when you are about to die. However well you wrap it up or present it, people still feel that when you go into such a place you will only come out 'feet first'. There is no denying that hospices and specialist palliative care units deal with death. There is no softening of that reality. It was to provide places where death could happen with dignity and care that was the stimulus for the creation of the modern hospice movement.

But we have to work hard at dispelling the perception that coming into a hospice is only about dying and the fact of death. Many patients, and the families who accompany them, carry with them on admission to a hospice profound levels of fear and anxiety about what it will be like and what it ultimately represents. Their understandable perception that it is a place only associated with death means they often expect it to be sombre and dull, that people will have to talk in whispers and walk on tiptoe, and that the only thing people will be talking about is death. To find brightness and laughter, a positive attitude, smiling faces, welcome and encourage-

ment does much to alter the perceptions and so dispel the initial fears
and anxieties. That is not to say there are not other kinds of fears
which arise as the journey continues. It is simply that right at the
beginning ideas can be changed, fears dissolved, and different work
done as a result.

However, problems remain. We are working hard to help people
get past their initial perceptions by creating a positive environment.
We are constantly enhancing the 'living rather than dying' concept,
and communicating a depth of care to patients and families to help
deal with their natural fears. And yet there is still one area of anxiety
among families and carers which is hard to overcome.

Let me illustrate this by telling you about Jenny and her mother.
I first met Jenny when she accompanied her mother onto the ward
at the time of her mother's admission. Jenny's mother was a delightful lady in her early 70s, widowed many years before, who had struggled on with an ever more serious condition over a number of years.
She had been cared for at home, well supported by the Primary Care
medical services, and with important input from one of our Marie
Curie specialist palliative care nurses. Jenny, her only daughter and a
single woman living with her mother, was her main carer, having
given up her job in order to be the focus of the support her mother
needed.

I spoke with Jenny while the nurses were settling the mother in
bed, and they and the doctors were gathering the information necessary on a patient's admission to the ward. Jenny was naturally
anxious. Her mother's symptoms needed to be 'sorted' and so they
had been persuaded that a short-term admission to the in-patient
unit would be advisable. Jenny wasn't at all sure about all of this. So I
tried to help her feel at home, attempting to create an environment
for her which would help her to relax, to get over her natural apprehensions about being in a new place, getting to know more people,
wondering what would be done and how things would work out for

the mother whom she cared for so much. She was, quite naturally, somewhat distracted during our discussion, obviously keen to be back with her mother, to continue to give the reassurance and support which was important to them both. So, when the nurses and doctors were done, Jenny went to be with her mother, and there, for the time being, the matter rested.

I touched base with Jenny and her mother on a number of occasions over the next few days. The initial anxieties had been worked through, and the positive environment and caring attitude of the staff had done its job. Jenny was keen to have her mother home again. But, as the symptoms were proving more difficult to control than had at first been expected, it was clear that this would be a longer admission than had been planned. Indeed, after a week or so Jenny's mother began to deteriorate. And, as she did so, Jenny's anxieties reappeared, but this time in a different form. I suspect that it was because the initial work had been done well and Jenny therefore had come to trust our staff that she felt she could share her anxieties. But she began to express her distress in a new way.

As her mother's condition worsened, she was moved to a single room. I came on to the ward one morning to find Jenny outside her mother's room while the nurses were tending to her mother's needs. She was crying. I suggested we go to the sitting room for some privacy, but she declined, not wanting to move too far away so that she could be immediately available to return to her mother's side when the nurses were finished. But she was open in her distress, and obviously willing to talk.

I was surprised by the first thing she said. 'I've let my mother down,' she sobbed. How could this be? How could such a caring and devoted daughter feel in any way that she had failed her mother. I felt puzzled, and obviously looked puzzled too. So Jenny continued. 'I've let her down badly, you see. I promised that I would keep her at home. I promised her she would die in her own bed. I promised her

I would care for her to the end. And now I can't. She'll die here. She's too poorly to go home. I've let her down.'

There was no criticism in all of that of the care we were offering, or of the rightness of that care being continued in our specialist unit. But there was great self-criticism, and a huge amount of self-recrimination, that what had been promised by a daughter could not now be fulfilled. This was the beginning of a pathway of guilt, a crippling and tortuous journey of self-criticism that so often begins before death and which can become a huge and often unmanageable burden in the process of bereavement.

I understood. And out of my understanding I offered what consolation and comfort I could. I tried to reassure Jenny that this was a partnership of care: she played her part and we played ours. Together we were doing the best for her mother. Home would not have worked at this stage. She had not failed.

She heard me. But clearly she did not accept my reasoning. A promise had been made, and a promise had been broken. A bond had been entered into and the bond had been departed from. So, she had failed.

I suspect that had Jenny's mother been well enough to talk this through with Jenny and others, she would have helped dispel the guilt, reassuring a caring daughter that she had done her best – more than anyone could have expected – and that she had not failed. But that opportunity was not open to us, such had been the rapidity of the deterioration. So Jenny was left with her broken promise, which at this stage was for her very hard to bear.

Jenny's mother died that night. I never saw Jenny again. She never responded to our invitations to come back for bereavement support. So I do not know if my words of reassurance helped. I do not know how she has coped with the guilt.

But what I do know is that the image of a broken daughter, and the expressions of failure which had contributed to the brokenness, have never left me. In different ways they have manifested themselves in similar circumstances over the years, in the struggle of carers to come to terms with that delicate balance between care at home and the role of an institution like a hospice or hospital. I have spoken often with people like Jenny who struggle with guilt through what they see as unfulfilled promises and unfinished care. And I have heard on many occasions from other chaplains and health-care professionals that this scenario is not in the least uncommon.

So, how do we deal with that? I have begun do so with another picture, one which, had I thought about it at the time, I might have shared with Jenny, but which in recent times has begun to form in my mind and which I have begun to share tentatively with some carers and families. It's beginning to make sense – just beginning. So, on this occasion, in its relatively unformed state, I share this new picture with you.

Carers have a tough job. It's as if they are steering a great ship across a vast ocean. They know the ship well. Through years of relationships, intimate knowledge, shared parts of the journey, they know the person for whom they now have to care. And there have been times when the ocean has been rough, and the task of steering this ship through stormy seas has been almost impossible. Others have helped along the way. The task of managing this vast liner has been shared. But the responsibility to captain, to steer, to manage the ship on its journey, has always and ultimately been in the hands of the carer who has made the promise always to be there, to stick to the task no matter what.

So what now of the end of the journey, when circumstances necessitate other people, specialists, taking over the care? What now when decisions are made by others, when the new environment of an institution has to be dealt with, when the great ship is in other people's hands? What now when the captain is no longer in command on the bridge?

It is as if, it appears to me, this vast liner is coming into port, as if it is now necessary to offer the delicate and skilled manoeuvres of bringing her safely to berth. So what do we do? We send a pilot out on a small launch to come onto the bridge and guide the ship home. This is a pilot who knows the home waters, the subtleties of the tides and the width of the harbour entrance, a pilot whose skills and knowledge have been made available to captains of many other liners which have berthed in this harbour.

But does the pilot take over the ship? Does the pilot dismiss the captain from the bridge? Does the pilot say the ship has changed ownership? Not at all. The pilot is the skilled and knowledgeable guest, there to stand with the captain and make his or her knowledge of the home waters available. It is still the captain's ship. The bridge is still the captain's domain. But the pilot is there to bring the ship safely home.

It is simply because the pilot knows how to bring the ship into 'port after stormy seas' that the task can be done well. Perhaps then 'death after life will greatly please' because the journey to the final resting place of the great liner has been one of care and calmness and dignity.

That is what Jenny was struggling with, wanting to do her best in her mother's last days, not knowing how to trust the pilot and to see at the same time that the care of the ship was still hers. I hope that, even though I had no picture to share with Jenny at the time, something of the truth of what we were doing got through.

It is interesting – and I don't want to push the picture too far, but none the less the thought does come to mind – that even if Jenny's mother were to have died at home, bringing the great ship to rest in the home port when death came would have been equally problematic, because those final waters of the reality of death would have been just as unfamiliar as they were in the surroundings of our hospice. So then too, in her own home, Jenny would have needed the subtle touch and knowledge of the pilot who knew the home waters of the dying process, to bring the ship safely to its final berth when death eventually came. The only difference would have been that this would have happened at home rather than in an institution. The same reality would have remained – the ship would have needed a pilot, and the bridge would still have been Jenny's.

Jenny wanted 'no more worry and waiting and troublesome doubt' for her mother (as John Betjeman writes in one of his poems) because she loved her so much. But she needed also to find that for herself, to know that sharing the care was not to fail, but to do even better than she was able to do by herself.

Towards calmer waters

He was a very simple old sailor, the skipper of a small boat that was taking them to the Shetlands, and they were a young, lively party, actors and actresses from London on tour, going to do a night or two on the Islands. They were not above 'taking the mickey' a bit, and they thought his way of saying grace before meals very quaint and old-fashioned. However, before long a storm blew up, a really severe north-easter, and as the little ship began to pitch more and more violently, morale among the visitors got lower and lower. A small deputation went up to ask the Captain's opinion. 'Well,' he said, 'maybe we'll get through, and maybe we won't. I never remember such a storm.' The news was greeted with dismay down below, and finally another deputation went up to the bridge to ask whether perhaps the Captain would be so good as to come and say a prayer with the terrified passengers. His reply was simply: 'I say my prayers when it's calm; and when it's rough, I attend to my ship.'

Anon

So, I've attended to my ship,
and I've made it through the storm.
It's been rough, but I've made it.
Now, when it's calm,
help me to pray,
help me to trust.
For I know that in these calm waters
storms will still rage –

storms of uncertainty,
of broken promises,
of letting go …
So, in these tranquil waters,
in the stillness of a ship in its home berth,
I pray for peace,
peace for my ship
and peace for my restless heart,
that I might rest a while,
in the calmness and safety of home.

Six

A door between two rooms

Think, in this batter'd Caravanserai
Whose Doorways are alternate Night and Day
Edward Fitzgerald: The Rubaiyat of Omar Khayyam

Death has a thousand doors to let out life. I shall find one.
Philip Massinger: A Very Woman

In my early days as a hospice chaplain I found myself sitting at the bedside of an elderly man. Tommy was in his mid-seventies, and I had got to know him, his wife Jean and various family members very well over the three weeks he had been a patient with us. Tommy was a practising Christian, a Church elder, and a leading figure in his local community. He was an intelligent man, quick-witted and good-humoured, and he loved good conversation – from the political events of the day to the varying fortunes of his favourite football team, from which of the nurses he fancied most to the state of the roses in the hospice garden.

Above all, Tommy loved to talk about his family: Jean his wife for 49 years, three wonderful daughters, four adored grandchildren, and a host of other relatives in the interconnecting circles of family life.

One thing he would not talk about, however, was his illness. He always appeared to me to be at peace with himself, with his loved ones and with his God – he was 'sorted' as my children would say. But, from time to time, I would give him the opportunity to talk things over, to check out whatever issues might be around of anxiety and fear. Each time he would give me clear signals, both verbal and non-verbal, that he would rather talk about other things. And talk he most certainly did – and I enjoyed his conversation-filled company very much.

On one particular occasion with Tommy I was in 'checking out mode', gently giving him the opportunity to talk about things that might need further sorting. Indeed, I had been asked to do just that by Tommy's consultant. She had informed me that morning that Tommy's recent batch of test results were not at all good, indicating that his cancer was galloping along faster than anyone had expected. She had talked with Tommy earlier in the day about the results, and had outlined as clearly as possible what the likely prognosis was – and it wasn't good. Tommy, she told me, had listened in an apparently uninterested fashion, had asked no questions, and appeared not to be disturbed at all by this latest bad news.

What was happening? she wondered. Had he heard her? Had he taken in what she had said? Had he switched off? Didn't he understand? Perhaps I could check it out and, from my knowledge of and relationship with Tommy, ascertain what might be going on in his mind.

So, there I was at Tommy's bedside, my mind full of the task in hand, prepared for questions and explorations. Tommy greeted me with a smile. 'Ah, the very man,' he exclaimed. 'I need a word.' This is it, I thought, the moment when he needed to open up – and I was ready for this moment. But his next sentence brought me crashing down to earth. 'I've been thinking about my Golden Wedding. I know it's nine months away, but we need to get organised. Jean'll not talk about it, so maybe you can help. Now, I've been thinking about the hall, and the band, and the guest list. And I think it would be nice if my minister was there, perhaps to say a blessing on our marriage. What do you think?' And in an instant I was drawn into Tommy's Golden Wedding plans, and we were comparing notes on venues and ceilidh bands, working out what the menu might be, planning the seating arrangements, and even talking through what kind of blessing he and Jean might have.

Through it all, Tommy was animated, enlivened, smiling broadly. This was a man who'd been told he had weeks, not months, to live. And here was a man sharing his Golden Wedding plans – for an event that was nine months hence.

What was I to do? Was I to interrupt and bring him back to the matter in hand ? Was I to say? 'Now look, Tommy, this is daft. You know and I know that you'll never see your Golden Wedding. So what's the point of all of this?' No, I don't think so. My task was to let Tommy live, and at that moment it was the planning of his Golden Wedding that allowed Tommy to live life to the full. My role was to go with Tommy into that 'lighted room' and enjoy the company of and celebration with people he loved.

Tommy died ten days later, with his plans for his Golden Wedding scribbled on the back of an envelope in his locker drawer – a clear indication if ever there was one that Tommy had lived until he died.

What was happening with Tommy? And what is happening to the many people we work with in our hospices who deal with things in similar ways?

It is clear that in the face of bad news and the reality of the prospect of death some people go into denial. But, in my experience, to label all those who take Tommy's approach as people in denial of reality is to categorise them in too simplistic a fashion. Even worse, it might incline us as carers to feel somewhat 'obliged' to pull them out of what we perceive to be their denial state.

Instead, I prefer to see it this way. In Tommy's head, and, I believe, in the inner recesses of the minds of all who are staring death in the face, there are two rooms with a connecting door. In one room there is the actuality, the facts clearly explained and, I believe more often than not, equally clearly understood. There is the prognosis, the medical terminology, the knowledge of death, the pain of separation, the sorrow that there will be an end to a finite life. And, on the other side of a flimsy wall and through a swinging connecting door, there is another room, of living, of 'normality', of planning Golden Weddings and the like.

Tommy had visited his room which contained the fact of his death. The consultant had done her job. The geography of that room had been clearly mapped out. And that had been enough for Tommy. He needed now to let the door swing closed and live in the room which was about living. He needed to keep the door closed between the two rooms for his own purposes of coping. That is not about denial. It is about conscious choice. It is about choosing to live as completely as possible for as long as that was likely.

What was living about for Tommy? It was about planning his Golden Wedding, of course, and filling that lighted room with hope and purpose, with laughter and smiles, with people he loved still.

I have no doubt at all that in his own way and in his own time Tommy would swing open the door between the two rooms, maybe just a crack, perhaps open wide, and gaze upon the reality of death, and check out the contents of that room once again. And I am equally sure that he would be right to close the door when he was done, again in his own time and for his own reasons, and go on living in the room of hope and life.

There would come a time for Tommy when there would be no choice left, when the adjoining door would be flung open, the flimsy wall torn down, the two rooms becoming one. There would be a time when for Tommy living with the reality of death would become part of the reality of life. But only Tommy would know when that time came for him. No one else might be privy to the moment or how he coped with it.

I use this image a lot with families. I do so not to cover over the need to explore sharing and talking, finishing the business and dealing with the healing of relationships and the like, but to explain what I see happening in people, to help us move from the labelling of 'denial' to the celebration of life and living.

Perhaps this is seen most clearly in the way children deal with death. I was asked by a mother of three small children who had been divorced from the children's father – a patient of ours, a man in his late thirties who had a brain tumour – to talk with her about the way the oldest of the three girls, aged nine, was coping with the prospect of her father's death. As a mother with what appeared to me to be an excellent relationship with her children, she had been very open with the girls who, despite the divorce, had remained close to their father. The three girls were, she explained, bright, interested and intelligent children. She had explained to them how ill their daddy was, that soon he would die, and that there was nothing the doctors could do to make their daddy better. The girls had been to visit their dad, had participated in his care, and had told him they loved him.

The worry was, however, how the eldest was coping. She seemed to be asking lots of questions one minute, and appearing uninterested the next. She would go from tears and distress to laughing uproariously at her favourite TV cartoon. She would switch in and out of seriousness and sorrow and questioning.

What was happening? her mother wondered. Was she OK? Had she, her mother, done anything wrong? What more should she be doing to make this journey of death manageable for her daughter?

I explained that switching in and out of grief, both before and after a death, was quite normal and healthy for a child. We do it as adults too. It's what Kahlil Gibran, when he reflects on joy and sorrow in his book *The Prophet*, describes as 'Your joy is your sorrow unmasked', and goes on to say:

And the selfsame well from which your laughter rises was oftentimes filled with your tears. And how else can it be? The deeper that sorrow carves into your being, the more joy you can contain. Is not the cup that holds your wine the very cup that was burned in the potter's oven? And is not the lute that soothes your spirit the very wood that was hollowed by knives? When you are joyous, look deep into your heart and you shall find it is only that which has given you sorrow that is now giving you joy. When you are sorrowful, look again in your heart and you shall see that in truth you are weeping for that which has been your delight. Some of you say 'Joy is greater than sorrow,' and others say, 'Nay, sorrow is the greater.' But I say to you they are inseparable. Together they come, and when one sits alone with you at your board, remember that the other is asleep on your bed. Verily you are suspended like scales between your sorrow and your joy. Only when you are empty are you at standstill and balanced. When the treasure keeper lifts you to weigh his gold and silver, needs must your joy or your sorrow rise or fall.

But somehow we as adults don't think it 'right' to laugh when we 'should' be crying. I was told once by a patient that when his mother died the minister had come to call in the middle of a bout of old-fashioned family laughter, and no one knew how to handle it because they thought the minister might deem it inappropriate or disrespectful. The poor man was reduced to having to go to his bedroom to bury his head in his pillow to stifle the laughter while his wife busied herself making the minister the obligatory cup of tea!

So with these thoughts and ideas in my mind, I used with that concerned mother the image of the rooms, making it clear that her daughter knew perfectly well what one room contained, and would look into it from time to time to check out the reality. But no one could expect a child to inhabit that room all the time. So she lived in the room filled with cartoons and pop music, with pals and school, with laughter and the normality of family life, and with a daddy still alive. One day there would be no door between the rooms. Reality would have to be faced. A nine-year-old would have no choice. But that would be 'one day'. This was now. There was another room to live in for the moment.

The mother nodded. She smiled. 'Now I understand,' she said. 'So it's my task to understand her when she peeps into the room she's closed the door on and help her interpret what she sees, and not to worry about how she's handling the balance between that and the rest of her life.' Goodness! She'd got it clearly, right enough. The reassurance for a caring mother was complete.

If Tommy's 'other' room was his Golden Wedding, should it not be our task, as well as helping him interpret the reality of death, also to celebrate with him the joy of living? And who is to say that it wasn't the Golden Wedding plans scribbled down on the back of an envelope, more than any other facet of our care and attention on the journey to death, that allowed Tommy to die with dignity and at peace?

Let me look

Let me look
and let me know again what lies
on the other side.

Let me flip the coin
and see the spinning sides of sorrow – joy,
joy – sorrow, sorrow – joy,
and know again
whatever side may fall
another side awaits.

Let me know again what I have always known
that the tapestry of this life
is not woven with a single thread –
no drabness here,
but life
with all its colours
in living richness.

Let me look again and know
the pain that has to be,
the loss
the sorrow
the death.

Let me look
and let me know what lies
on the other side.

And let me turn again
and laugh
and shout afresh with children

and sing anew with those who know my songs;
and let me turn again and know
the other side
as if I were seeing it for the first time,
and fall in love,
and hold my child,
and feel at one with God.

Let me turn again and know
that this is life,
the whole of life.

Let me turn again and live with this
and know what life contains
in all its fullness.

Then let me look
and let me know what lies
on the other side.

But tell me not to stay,
but turn again
and know again
that this is life,
and this is death,
and both are one.

And let me choose to turn to that which is my living,
till all is one,
and death and living
are Living again,
and dying is no more.

I have a friend whose prayer-life is all about doors! Every time he passes through a door, at work, at home, with friends, at leisure, he prays for what he has left behind – the people, the circumstances, his contribution, his failings – and what he is about to deal with – new situations, people to be helped, work to be done, and the like. He even tells me it works when he goes to a football match or to the shops!

Why not give it a try? And, as you do so, the prayers on the page opposite might be helpful.

A prayer on leaving

This has been your place, Lord,
and I have shared it with you for a time.
As I have known you there,
may you remain known to those who stay.
When I have neglected you there,
be patient with those who may neglect you now.
Let your healing love fill that place,
that those who come and go as I have done,
might be ever aware that they share this place with you.

A prayer on entering

This is your place, Lord.
You have been here long before I came along.
You will be with me for as long as I stay.
Let me not feel that all that happens here is in my hands alone,
to heal and to help, to direct and control,
but let me trust in your way and in your wisdom,
for all that is yet to be.

Seven

Clearing the attic

Put everything in order because you will not recover. Get ready to die.
Isaiah 38:1

Make it your aim to live a quiet life, to mind your own business, and to earn your own living, just as we told you before.
I Thessalonians 4:11

Within the fields of health care and social welfare, and particularly in palliative medicine, there is a clear commitment to holistic care, a focus on all aspects of well-being – physical, psychological, social, emotional and spiritual. Amongst this range of needs, the spiritual dimension deserves equal recognition and attention.

Yet despite all that has been written about spiritual care in recent years, there remains for many an inadequate understanding of its meaning. As a consequence, too little attention is given to spiritual issues in professional training. It is no surprise, therefore, that the commitment to spiritual care sometimes leaves much to be desired in practice.

However spiritual care is defined – and there are many definitions in current use – there is a clear move towards understanding it as a desire to find purpose and fulfilment or, as I have said in an earlier chapter, as a search for meaning, faith and hope, and a recognition of the wholeness and value of life.

All of us, all of the time, are engaged in this searching process in one way or another, consciously and subconsciously. Most of us get by without giving such big issues a lot of thought. But for those who are dying, with time rapidly running out, the need to focus on them often becomes acute. In my experience what people concentrate on in the face of death is not the life that is to come – whether they understand that concept in a religious or humanist framework – but the nature of the life they are about to leave behind. It is for this that they need to find meaning, purpose and fulfilment before it comes to an end.

The image which helps me in this instance is one that I have used a lot in explaining the nature of spiritual care and in understanding what people are searching for in the face of death. Indeed it is a picture which was formative for me as a hospice chaplain and which has been of greatest use in my understanding of my needs and the needs of others as we work together with their issues. And it is a picture I got from William.

William was 54 years old, single, lived alone, and was dying of cancer. He had been referred by his GP to our home care service, and one of our specialist palliative care nurses called to see him at home. He would not let her in, and sent her away with a flea in her ear! So, all we knew about William was his name, address and date of birth, where he lived and what his diagnosis was. And there we had to let the matter rest.

One day, quite out of the blue, William appeared at our Centre and asked 'to see the boss'. Having identified him as the patient who had been referred to us some weeks before, our Medical Director sat down with him to talk, and William expressed his purpose in seeking out the boss. 'I need some help,' he said, 'to clear out my mental attic before I die.' In the discussion which ensued, William was offered a number of resources – social worker, doctor, home care sister, chaplain – to help him clear out his attic. William chose the chaplain. Why he did so, I do not know. I can only surmise. But the next day, following a telephone contact to arrange a convenient time, he and I met for the first time.

Once we had gone through the niceties of the tea and biscuits, I was quite unprepared for his opening gambit. 'When I was told that

I had cancer,' he began, 'I set aside an evening for myself to work out the answers to two questions: Firstly – am I religious? And secondly – do I believe in God? After much heart-searching, I decided that my answer to both questions was no. Now, chaplain, is that a problem for you?' 'No,' I replied. 'It's not a problem at all. And now that we've got that out of the way, what help do you need to clear out your mental attic?'

Over four afternoons, a week apart and an hour-and-a-half each time, William laid bare the dark corners of his attic – and it was extensive and very messy. Issues of guilt, broken relationships, his struggle with being gay, childhood rejections, his lack of self-worth, what his will might contain, his fears for his alcoholic friend, and much more, were carefully explored. We even talked about his funeral. (He wanted a huge firework display, I recall, 'the kind they have at the end of the Edinburgh Festival'. But he had discovered that to have such a display required clearance from Air Traffic Control at Edinburgh Airport because it could disrupt the aircraft flight-paths. So they needed to know the date and the time of the firework display. And it wasn't possible to predict that! So he'd had to adjust his plans.)

There was much in William's attic which needed clearing. And though time was short, William was not to be rushed, and sought to deal with each issue, each tidying process, carefully and thoroughly. Eventually, to his satisfaction, the job was completed. At the end of our final session together, he thanked me for my time. The attic was in order. I wouldn't see him again. And he and I wished each other well. To this day, I do not know what happened to William. He will have died a long time since. But I do know that the task William had set himself was completed, and because of that he was at peace.

This image of clearing the untidy attic is a powerful one, and I don't think I have ever come across someone who has been so focused on the task of clearing it out. William was, I believe, a spiritual being clearly engaged in a spiritual search – despite his protestations about being non-religious. As he struggled to find meaning for his complicated life – to tidy his attic before he died – he was going to the core of his being, seeking meaning, purpose and fulfilment. That is fundamental to the human condition. And it is spiritual!

Meister Eckhart wrote:

A man has many skins in himself, covering the depths of his heart. Man knows so many things; he does not know himself. Why, thirty or forty skins or hides, just like an ox's or a bear's, so thick and hard, cover the soul. Go into your own ground and learn to know yourself there.

I have no doubt that before he died, having stripped away layers of covering in this spiritual search, William somehow succeeded in finding his soul, and went into his own ground and learned to know himself – perhaps for the very first time.

We are all spiritual beings. Spirituality is so hard to define that it is often labelled as esoteric, dismissed as peripheral, or seen as the pursuit only of the high-minded. And yet, if holistic care includes the spiritual dimension, to dismiss it or avoid it is to do an injustice to the person for whom we care. William knew that, and therefore in seeking purpose and fulfilment for his life before he died he was on a spiritual journey, moving towards being a whole person.

In his case, he needed help. His attic was too scary a place to venture into alone after all those years, and too messy by far. Many who seek to make sense of life in the face of death have few, if any, resources within themselves, of language, symbols or beliefs, upon which they can draw. It is our task as carers to help them find these resources to finish their task.

The job William needed to do could not and should not be confined to a religious framework. He had no belief in a divine being and he was not a religious man. And yet he still had a spiritual search. And this, for some, is a problem. From the 'religious' side there is the misconception that religion alone defines spirituality and only the religious are spiritual people; and from the 'secular' side there is the naive assumption that religion and spirituality are synonymous. William had ditched concepts of God and religion. He also knew I was a religious man. But to begin his search, it was necessary for William to be affirmed where he was – and that was in his attic and not mine.

If we are to be genuine with people in their spiritual search, then sometimes concepts of God have to be left to one side. Religion does not work for everyone, and God does not have to be imposed on every facet of spiritual care. You can ask people like William!

If it is true that it is most unhelpful to stand on our city walls and shout advice to the lost traveller and make no attempt to meet them in their desert (to use an image from an earlier chapter), then to stand beneath the trap-door of William's attic and shout instructions, when we are not with him and know nothing of his fears and anxieties, is equally unhelpful. But worse, to stand at the door of our own house, where we suppose our religious attic is neat and tidy, and persuade William to come and be where we are, is uncaring. For if William did come to our house, there would be so much unfinished business left behind in his attic that he might face death with greater anxiety and fear.

The advantage of the 'search for meaning' approach to spiritual care is that it takes people seriously, for it contains an understanding that all people have spiritual needs, and in dealing with them the focus is on helping people find their own meaning rather than the carers sharing their faith.

Until we fully grasp this approach, is it any wonder that the caring professions remain suspicious of spiritual care if they have a false concept of it? And is it any wonder that spiritual care is neglected in professional training if it is assumed that you have to be religious to give and receive a grounding in spiritual issues?

If the dying person has had time and help to tidy their attic before they die, might they not then be able to live at peace and with quality of life in their house right to the very end?

While I speak within the context of working as a chaplain in a Marie Curie Centre, all who work in health and social care have to grasp the reality of these issues. We must understand William's basic principles – that spirituality is common to all, and that it is not always synonymous with religion. And we must go on to weave an understanding of spiritual care into the fabric of all professional training and development. Then, and only then, can we say we are truly holistic in our approach.

It is our task to help people be clear about the essence of their being. And whatever the essence is, whatever the messy attic contains, it is that which needs healing, sorting out, before death comes. And it is there we must begin.

But a word of warning, the same warning which would apply with the picture of the desert and sharing the tears. When you enter into an attic which is in the state William's was in, you can't help but get a little messed up too. Some of the dust will cling, some of the fears will be disturbing, some of the sorrow will touch you deeply. Some of your own attitudes will be challenged. You cannot fully be in the attic without it affecting you.

Avoidance of that fact – to take William away from his attic into your own house, or to stay outside his attic and shout instructions for his tidying – is not only to be of little help to William, but is to keep you aloof, separate, immune from his pain. To be with him, fully with him, is bound to affect you deeply too.

So, when you leave the attic, you have to dust yourself down in order to stay healthy – to be debriefed, to get help, to find super-vision, to have spiritual direction, or whatever.

Indeed, you might be challenged by what you have done in William's attic to look at some issues you need to sort out in your

own, and you may need help to do that, just as you helped William.
You may, in your time, say to someone else: 'I need help to clear out
my attic ...' That is real and it is healthy. It is about growth and
development. And it is also about being able to leave your house day
after day with the capacity to enter into more attics and help others
do the tidying, knowing that you can come home afterwards and
find renewed peace and regeneration in your own house.

I recently conducted the funeral of a 32-year-old wife and
mother who died in our hospice. She was a most delightful woman,
and had a wonderful husband, good family support, and two lovely
little children. As part of her funeral service her husband asked me to
read out something he had written, a personal reflection on what he
had learned as he and his wife faced illness and the prospect of death.
It was a brave thing to offer in public his personal thoughts. But he
believed it to be right. With his permission I quote part of what he
wrote, and you will see, with me, how right it was.

*If I've learned any lessons from this tragic and painful past few months it is
that life itself is very fragile and one shouldn't assume that they will automatically live a long life. Make the most of life because you never know when
it will be taken away from you – live life to the full every day – not just occasionally. If you love someone, tell them so and don't assume they know,
because one day a time will come when they won't be there to tell any more.*

In these deep and beautiful words a young husband and father
showed that something of his attic had been cleared. Some 'stuff' had
been 'sorted'. And the attics of relationships and how we deal with
each other have to keep being 'sorted' so that living can go on being
fulfilling.

In so doing, and in offering his words for me to read out, he was
asking me if there were things in my attic which needed tidying –
people I needed to say 'sorry' to, someone I needed to write to, a love
taken for granted I needed to express again.

What is it in my house and in my attic that needs to be looked at again so that my house gives me the regeneration I need? Who do I need to help with my tidying? Shouldn't I get on with it in case 'one day a time will come' when it is simply too late?

To rest

It's been a tough day.
I don't know why I have to care so much,
but I do.
So I care so much
it hurts,
and it costs,
and it drains me of my life.

So, I'm home,
now,
at last,
to rest with you.

Let me feel your warmth
in my glass of wine;

let me feel your healing touch
as my body relaxes in a warm bath;

let me feel your stimulation
as I struggle with a crossword clue;

let me sense your wisdom
as I lose myself in a good book;

let me know your joy
as I laugh and cry with a comedy show;

let me feel my worth
as the phone rings

and the machine answers it
and I don't care for now;

let me feel your renewal
as I'm kissed with loving lips;

let me feel re-created
in the presence of good friends;

let me feel your insight
as I write in my journal;

let me feel holy
as I feel your holiness;

let me be challenged and prompted
by what I am learning about me;

let me be renewed as I sleep.

It's been a tough day.
But I'm home,
for me,
with you,
so that I might learn to care again
and love again
and give again
to others,
and to me,
and to you.

God of my home

God of my home,
thank you for rest and security,
for family and friendships,
for life and for love.

God of my tidy rooms,
thank you for purpose and reason,
for faith and hopefulness
for order and peace.

God of my cries for help,
hear me in my confusion and my yearnings
my honesty and my searching,
my broken dreams and unfulfilled desires.

God of my messed up life,
be with me in my struggles and turmoil,
my sorting and my discarding
my tears and my weariness.

God of my unfinished tasks,
help me with the ragged edges and incompleteness,
what I know in part and finish in part,
in my faith and life.

God of my resting,
comfort me in my letting go and my leavings,
my endings and my departings,
that I might know that I have done enough for now.

God of this, my home,
thank you for what's down here and what's up there,
the known and the unknown,
the sure and the uncertain,
the completed and the newly begun,
of my home and Yours.

Eight

The broken contract

All sensible people are selfish, and nature is tugging at every contract to make the terms of it fair.
Ralph Waldo Emerson: Conduct of Life

My God, my God, why have you abandoned me?
Psalm 22:1

When spiritual care is considered as an integral part of the holistic process of caring for people, it should be no surprise that the Williams of this world pop up from time to time and challenge preconceptions about what is being offered. It may be a surprise to many, and indeed it may be disturbing to some, that spiritual care can be offered to and can work for the atheist. But that is the fact. It is, if you like, the clearing of the attic that matters not the location of the house.

It is from the other end of the spectrum, however, that another – though not unrelated – issue arises, which in many ways is even more challenging and threatening, certainly to those who hold strongly to a framework of faith and a set of religious beliefs and practices. It leads to a picture which, to be honest, I don't like much, but which I have felt it important to struggle with and make sense of in the field of spiritual care and my day-to-day work as a chaplain. But first let me explain how it arose.

Violet was 63 years old. She had tumour-related spinal cord compression, and was living with a slowly developing paralysis. As an in-patient for an extended period of time, she was worked with and cared for by all members of our team and, in terms of relationships, by some more successfully than others.

She had five grown-up children, and her husband had died several years before. The family situation was tense, as individuals within it struggled in their own way to cope with Violet's increasing disability, her times of depression, and her increasingly demanding nature.

Violet was not an easy person to care for. There was so much anger and frustration around that she often presented herself as being unaccepting and uncooperative.

She was also a very religious woman, a practising Christian, and a regular attender at her local church. She was what could be described as a 'pillar' of her congregation – Sunday School teacher when she was younger, prayer-meeting organiser, old-people visitor, and much more – an all-round good Christian lady.

And Violet was frightened of dying. Not only that, but the faith by which she had lived, the relationship she had built up with her God, the religious structure in which she had felt comfortable for so long had, to her mind, all failed her. And all attempts to help her re-interpret God and faith had failed too. Indeed, the bottom line was that God had failed his loving servant. The God in whom she had put her trust had broken his part of the deal she in faith had made with him – whereby she would live a good life and God for his part would keep her alive, or at least keep her from suffering and having bad feelings about death. And she had lived a good life. She had kept her part of the bargain. But now she was going to die, and the dying was going to be painful and debilitating, and she was very scared, and very, very angry. This was God's fault. He had failed her. She had been conned. It was as if her contact of faith, her contact with God, had been broken.

In her distress, Violet turned to the chaplain, the religious man whom she trusted. This was the person whom she perceived as having the answers to help 'fix' the contract and make it work again.

I talked and shared at a very deep level with Violet. More than once I found myself in that 'Godless' desert where she so often languished, being dragged down into the faithless depression which threatened to overwhelm her. But I was not prepared to offer her the sticking-plasters of ready solutions for her faith which she so clearly demanded of me. I declined to take the role of the 'fixer'. Yet every time I sought to deal sincerely and openly with her dilemmas, including offering reflections on my own faith journey, interpretations of biblical passages and the hope of the Gospel, another issue would arise, another problem would come to the surface. If I did have sticking-plasters to offer, they would have run out at a very early stage! Violet was trapping me in the role of religious fixer and as such she would tell you I failed.

It was clear to me that bad religion and bad practices of ministers, priests and religious teachers had caused damage to this lady. They had created for her a dependence on someone else's knowledge, on someone else's certainty, and and had left her lacking in the skills needed for a genuine search for truth as it mattered to her.

As I worked with Violet, I became convinced that she needed to be freed from the concepts of God and religion which were crippling her, freed from an inability to see what needed to be done and said and worked with before she died. Faith for Violet was at the head level, only in the intellect. It had never become fully part of her, something integral to her whole being. One could say Violet's faith had never become a spiritual matter.

So, like William, she needed to ditch that kind of religion, or at least the concept of religion which had been built up and reinforced through many years – and clear out her mental attic too. She needed to be free to work on her spiritual issues. But, sadly, her religion did not allow her that freedom.

So she struggled on in her darkness, with her sense of failure, with God's failure to hold to his side of the contract, and with the failure of even the chaplain to fix things up for her and make her better. Perhaps she even saw the chaplain's failure as just another sign of God's failure. For, after all, wasn't he supposed to be God's representative?

If spiritual care is the healing of that inner part of our being which is dislocated in the face of death, and if someone like William can be seen as a spiritual being even though he is an atheist, might it not be the case that Violet too had to find that spiritual part of her being and recognise its brokenness and seek healing for it, and that she might have to begin to abandon her concept of religion to do so? Because, for Violet, faith – or, to be accurate, her interpretation of it – was getting in the way.

Now that is a bold assertion, and it in no way denies the value, worth and purpose which a faith structure gives a person, including myself, to deal with issues of living and dying. But that faith system only works when it is real, and it is only real when it is spiritual, and it only moves to the realms of the spiritual when religion is seen as a pathway to wholeness and not a destination in itself.

There is a cartoon strip called 'The Broons' in Scotland's much-read Sunday newspaper *The Sunday Post* which, week by week, depicts the antics of a large Scottish family. In one Sunday's edition, there was Maw Broon, the matriarchal head of the family, with a fancy iced cake, and the unfolding story showed how, person by person, the family tried to persuade her to share the cake around. But she was having none of it. The cake was too lovely, too precious to spoil. Eventually, however, the family's wishes prevailed and, with great ceremony and with the whole family gathered round, Maw Broon cut the cake. It was immediately clear that there was a major problem. For Maw Broon had taken so long to share the cake that a family of little mice had got in underneath, eaten all the cake itself, and left only the fancy icing. So, when the knife went it, the icing crumbled to dust on the table and there was nothing to share.

I have a sense sometimes that we allow, indeed we encourage, people to build their faith like the layers of fancy icing on a cake, so that it is beautiful to look at and a joy to behold. But if it has no substance, no earthy, solid, somewhat unattractive substance, when the knife of pain, loss, tragedy or doubt cuts in, there is nothing to absorb it, no 'body' of goodness to cut into, and the whole thing crumbles to dust in front of your eyes.

What we need to help people find is substance to faith, not fancy icing. What they need is earthiness, and not the creation of a thing of beauty.

Many people who are religious never have to face the problem Violet had. Indeed the majority of people who have a belief system find religion and God a great strength in the face of suffering and death. They have that solidity to begin to absorb the tragedy and pain and the knowledge of life's mortality. But for the few who are the Violets of this world even chaplains struggle to rescue them from years of bad religion and flawed concepts of God built up over a life-time with decoration and fancy style.

Violet's struggle with the broken contract with God never allowed her to find that spiritual preparation for death which could have been hers. That is sad, because it is possible for people to deal with all of this and find a renewed perspective on faith in the face of death which can also include, if you like, a revised contract with God.

The dying person, if the environment is right and there are the proper resources to help, needs to write their own script concerning death. To facilitate that, we need – out there in the big world of religions and religious ideas – to begin to reclaim the notion of a spiritual search and not assume that religious beliefs per se do it all for us.

I hope, and indeed I believe, that we got the environment right for Violet. But the process of reclamation somehow eluded her. It need not have done, because there is potential, I believe, for people to use the reality of their own death to find God again, and to be renewed deep within the soul.

I like this Hasidic tale told by Anthony De Mello:

One night Rabbi Isaac was told in his dream to go to faraway Prague and there to dig for hidden treasure under a bridge that led to the palace of the King. He did not take the dream seriously, but when it recurred four or five times, he made up his mind to go in search of the treasure. When he got to the bridge, he discovered to his dismay that it was heavily guarded day and night by soldiers. All he could do was gaze at the bridge from a distance. But since he went there every morning, the captain of the guards came up to him one day to find out why. Rabbi Isaac, embarrassed as he was to tell his dream to another soul, told the captain everything, for he liked the good-natured character of this Christian. The captain roared with laughter and said, 'Good heavens! You a Rabbi and you take dreams so seriously? Why, if I were stupid enough to act on my own dreams, I would be wandering around in Poland today. Let me tell you one I had last night that keeps recurring frequently: A voice tells me to go to Krakow and dig for treasure in the corner of the kitchen of one Isaac, son of Ezechiel! Now, wouldn't it be the most stupid thing in the world to search around Krakow for a man called Isaac and another called Ezechiel when half the male population there probably has one name and the other half the other?' The Rabbi was stunned. He thanked the captain for his advice, hurried home, dug up the corner of his kitchen, and found a treasure abundant enough to keep him in comfort till the day he died.

De Mello reminds us that the spiritual quest is a journey without distance. You travel from where you are right now to where you have always been. Eventually you come to see that what you think you are seeing for the first time is what has been right under your nose from the beginning.

We tried to make that possible for Violet. The journey she needed to travel was that short distance from the head to the heart.

The God she was looking for was already there. But, for her, even that short distance was too long to find the truth that was there all the time.

Spirituality, and in Violet's Christian framework the search for the true God, is a matter of becoming what you really are and finding the God who is really there. Violet's search never brought her back to herself, and did not allow her to find the enlightenment she needed – which could, indeed, have been so close at hand, and which would have given some renewed purpose to her life and her relationship with God.

De Mello illustrates this with another reflection:

A young man became obsessed with a passion for Truth, so he took his leave of his family and friends and set out in search for it. He travelled over many lands, sailed across many oceans, climbed many mountains, and, all in all, went through a great deal of hardship and suffering. One day he woke to find he was seventy-five years old and had still not found the Truth he had been searching for. So he decided, sadly, to give up the search and go back home. It took him months to return to his hometown for he was an old man now. Once home, he opened the door of his house – and there found that Truth had been patiently waiting for him all those years.

The journeying had not helped him find Truth, but it had prepared him to recognise it. In many ways the journey of Violet's faith had not been a journey but a conclusion, a finding of the Truth she sought. But it didn't work. Nor did she see that the journey could never be an end in itself, but that its purpose was to prepare her to find the Truth that had been waiting for her all the time.

Inevitably, as I work with people like Violet, and ponder my own inner doubts and fears, I have to ask myself searching questions about my own faith and my own trust in God. I don't always get it right. Nor am I ever absolutely sure about all aspects of faith. But I hope that I will keep working with the reality of where I am and what I feel, and like Jacob of old, not be afraid to wrestle with God and perhaps even limp away from the struggle.

Some years ago I had a holiday with my wife in St Andrew's. The weather was pretty miserable, so I decided to buy an umbrella – and what else could I do in the home of golf but buy a big golf umbrella in Gordon tartan. I was very pleased with my umbrella, and it certainly did its job in rainy St Andrew's. When I got back to Edinburgh, the first Sunday I was due to take the morning service in my church it was pouring with rain once more. But undaunted – and pleased with the opportunity to show off my new purchase to my congregation – I walked the ten minutes to church sheltering under my fine umbrella. Half way there, however, I realised I had a problem, not with the umbrella but with my right shoe which was letting in water at an alarming rate. By the time I reached the church I was bone dry from the ankles upwards, but my right foot was sopping wet.

Muttering under my breath about my misfortune, and shaking my foot to be rid of at least some of the dampness, I ascended the church steps to be greeted by Sandy, my Church Officer, with a big smile on his face. 'Nice umbrella!' he commented. 'But what's the point in having the best umbrella in the world if your shoes leak?'

What indeed? What's the point of being sheltered from above if down at ground level things just aren't working right? What's the point of all the faith you can muster if the basic stuff isn't sorted?

Sandy was right. Faith is fine, and the protection of the Love of God is so important to those who trust and believe. The old Irish hymn 'Be thou my vision' affirms for us: 'Thou my soul's shelter, thou my high tower: raise thou me heavenward, O power of my power' – and what purpose we do gain and shelter we do find in the power and presence of God! But aren't we also charged with the responsibility of working at the basics, the down-to-earth stuff of our daily living, so that we and God are working together on the journey through life's stormy days?

'God's in his heaven, all's right with the world' wrote Robert Browning. But do we find it so? I think not – at least, not all the time. And Violet certainly didn't. So, what's the point in having the best umbrella in the world if your shoes leak? Where is the purpose of faith if we don't do our bit too?

God?

This reflection was written down immediately following an interaction with a distraught husband and father who was hours away from the death of his wife at the age of thirty-two, leaving behind her two beautiful little children. This man was a devout Christian, and in his anguish was fundamentally honest about his under-standing of God. His pain became my pain, and so these words are a powerful reflection of how we both felt at the time. I offer them to you out of his honesty and mine.

'Your God is a bastard!' he screamed.
My God?
My God!
Was he right?

Eloi, Eloi, lema sabachthani
(A reflection on Psalm 22:1–5)

My God, my God, why have you abandoned me?
My God!
My God?
But were you mine
when I knew you
and loved you
and held you
and blessed you?
Or were you some illusion,
some trick
some fake
to leave me now
wondering
and waiting
for you to come again?

I have cried desperately for your help.
You bet, I've cried.
You know I've cried –
with anger
and with tears.
I have wept in your absence
and my impotence.
I have hoped
and prayed
and longed for your reassuring touch.
But still it does not come.

During the day I call to you
but you do not answer.

Are you asleep?
Did I choose the wrong time?
Are you too busy?
Have you gone away?
Or is it me?
Don't you like me,
listen to me
care for me any more?
During the day,
and all night,
all the long, dark night
I call,
but I get no rest from my turmoil
no rest from your response,
no peace.

But …
you are up there,
I know you are,
enthroned
in glory.
We've been saying that for years
in worship
in creeds
in praise.
Our ancestors put their trust in you.
They trusted you.
You were OK for them –
you touched them,
you healed them,

you comforted them,
you believed in them
as much as they believed in you.

You listened when they called.
You took them out of danger.
They trusted you
and they weren't disappointed.

So what about me?
Why can't I be as sure as them,
as trusting as them
as believing as them?
Why can't I know
that you will save me from my danger too?

God, I'm waiting.
I want to know you'll come.
I want to believe
I'll believe in you again.

Eloi, Eloi,
My God, my God,
Have you abandoned me?
Why?
My God, my God,
Come to me now …

What now, God?

I signed my name, Lord,
I took the plunge; I gave my all.
What now, of life and love?
What now of God for me?

I made my choice, Lord,
I nailed my colours to your mast.
What now, of worth and value?
What now of God for me?

I offered life, Lord,
the life I had, the only life I knew.
What now, or life and living?
What now of God for me?

'I gave my name, child,
to be "I Am" for you, to make you as I am.
This now is life and love.
This, now, is God in you.

'I made my choice, choice,
for I chose you, unique in all the world.
You now are worth and value.
This, now, is God for you.

'I gave my Life, child,
that you might live and know what living means.
And you are living proof
that, now, God lives for you.'

I do not know, Lord, what I should do, or think, or say.
What now, of prayers and faith?
What now of God for me?

'I do not know, child, what I should do.
Only I stretch my arm and take your hand.
This is my faith, my love; this – now – of God for you.'

Nine

Finishing the business

The charter of thy work gives thee releasing.
William Shakespeare: Sonnet

It is finished.
John 19:30

There is no doubt that the people who cope best as they face the knowledge of their own death, and the people who cope best with the process of bereavement after their loved one has died, are those who, before death comes, have taken time to finish the business. One such man was Bobby, who taught me much about the necessity to make sense of a life before it could be let go, and about the need for an unconditional affirmation of the worth of that life.

Bobby was 72 years old, and he was dying of lung cancer. When he was admitted to our hospice for control of his pain, two things quickly became clear. Firstly, this was likely to be a 'continuing care' admission as Bobby was a very sick man; and, secondly, this was not going to be an easy man to work with, such was his aggression and uncooperative nature.

Bobby had done little to endear himself to the nursing team during the first 24 hours of his admission. He had been aggressive, uncompliant, foul-mouthed, and extremely chauvinist to and dismissive of the young nurses. When I met him, he was on his own in one of our sitting rooms, crumpled in a big easy-chair. He looked grey, and he was puffing on a very thin roll-up cigarette. 'Hello, my name's Tom and I'm the chaplain here. How're you doing?' I said, offering my hand. He took it – reluctantly – and pronounced, with all the endearing passion his weak frame could muster, 'You'd be as well buggerin' off, son. There's nae point in talkin' tae me. See, 'am a Marxist and an atheist masel'. So you can bugger off and bother someone else with your religion.' If I'd been quick enough, I'd have said something clever or witty. But I wasn't. So I simply said, 'I just wanted to say hello. I'll catch you another time.' And I hoped I wouldn't have to bother.

The next day there was a message for me in the nurses' Duty Room: 'Bobby wants to see you – in the sitting room – at 10 o'clock – sharp!' I was intrigued and not a little apprehensive when I went to meet Bobby for the second time. And I found him as I had done the day before, in a big chair, drawing hard on another roll-up. But this time the atmosphere was distinctly different. He saw me come in, and said, 'Aye, right son, come in. Sit yersel' down' – as if it was his front room – 'Now, how long've you got?' I replied, 'As long as you need. But why?' 'Because I dinnae want ye tae run away. I want tae tell ye ma life story.'

And he did – from the age of thirteen when he first went down the pit (having lied about his age so he could get a job in order to supplement the meagre income of a large, fatherless family), his Catholic upbringing, becoming a Communist at sixteen, through years of capitalist exploitation, union politics, family stresses, picket-lines, Arthur Scargill, Mick McGahey, the 'wicked witch Thatcher', ministers and priests he'd known through the years, drink, smoking, religion, friendships, the prospect of death, the lot! It took him an hour and a half. It was arduous for him. And when he was done, he slumped back exhausted in his chair. There was a long silence. After a while he leaned forward and said quietly: 'Well, son, what do you make o' that?' 'What do you mean, "what do I make of that"?' I asked. (I knew full well what he meant, but I'd long ago picked up the skill of answering a question with a question because it gives you time to think of an answer. Ask my children!) Bobby sighed. 'You know, son. Has my life been any good? Will it do?'

At that moment I believe a craggy old miner was asking a spiritual question. And why of someone with whom he would never agree in religious terms? Because of ministers and priests he had known through his life whom he respected because they had stood with miners on picket-lines when it was not socially or ecclesiastically acceptable to do so. He respected my 'label' and I respected his. And he was prepared to meet in the middle.

'Yes,' I replied, 'it'll do! A life's work for better conditions for miners, facing social injustice head on? That'll do for me.'

Bobby died a week or so later, and with a greater peace and considerably less anger than he had shown on admission. More people than I played their part in that. But I know Bobby was on a spiritual journey, sorting things out before he died, finishing the business, concluding a search for meaning, purpose, fulfilment, and perhaps above all finding an affirmation of the worth of his life.

In hospices we seek to deal with the whole person, not just the part of them which is their cancer. So, if we are to achieve the best quality of life for each person, the spiritual dimension is important. And for Bobby the spiritual dimension was about finishing the business before he died.

A hospice setting acknowledges patients in their uniqueness. Now that there is considerable expertise in relieving physical symptoms, there is the opportunity to explore the spiritual needs of dying people. However, whilst the physical, emotional and social components are reasonably clearly understood, the spiritual domain, as I have indicated before, is far less well defined.

And that is a problem. It is hard to define the spiritual. Everyone experiences a challenge and dislocation in the face of death. Bobby taught me that. He found himself physically, mentally and spiritually dislocated to a place he had not been in before – the journey to death. And that was scary! But the value of spiritual care was that in that dislocation he was supported in his search for meaning, and he was able to begin to make sense of the whole of life before he died.

But this brings us once again to a difficulty we have already touched upon. Because spirituality is so hard to define, it is very often confused with religion.

The spiritual search happens inside and outwith a framework of religious beliefs. Some people will have spiritual needs and no religious needs. If, as I have indicated, everyone has a need for meaning in life, some who are interested in God and religion will work through these channels to find their meaning and purpose. But others cannot or will not. They may have been exposed to religion in younger years, may even have been confirmed, but have rejected religious beliefs and practices in adult life simply because they do not make sense any more. In addition, more and more people in our present society have never been exposed to religious beliefs and practices at all and have, therefore, never even thought about what religion might entail.

So, for many and, indeed, perhaps even for most, the process of meaning is explored in different directions, such as art, music, politics, work, philosophy and the like. For Bobby it was Marxism which had given him meaning all his life. So to confine the essence of being to a religious framework alone, and worse, to insist that people are dragged into a religious framework before they die, is to fail to recognise other frameworks which give people meaning and define for them their spiritual search.

Bobby's spiritual question was, 'Has my life been any good?' If I had replied, 'Well, no. The only way we can really say it's been good is if you "get religion". The only way to heaven is ...' or something of the sort, if I hadn't already had a roll-up stubbed out on my thigh, I would have been told to, 'Bugger off with your religion, son!'... and the moment of healing and affirmation would have been lost. It was my task to be Bobby's companion, to travel with him on his spiritual journey, not to insist he travel on mine.

It is the personal and unique meaning that patients associate with their own spirituality which is important, and our response to their desire to 'finish the business' within that framework which is vital. The atheist and the agnostic will look outwith the concept of God for a framework to work with. But in terms of a search for meaning, a framework, and the finishing of their business within it, is just as vital as for believers. Bobby was a Marxist and atheist. I am a Christian minister and a hospice chaplain. But in a hospice sitting room we shared a spiritual journey together, so that life had meaning – for both of us – in the face of death.

In telling Bobby's story – as I have done many times over the years – I have often been asked if I have a right to define what I believed was happening to him in my terms – using the language of spirituality – when, clearly, he would never have defined it in such a way. Yes, I believe I do, because that is my framework, my way of understanding, explaining, being excited by the mystery that was Bobby's search. So I say and I believe that Bobby experienced spiritual care in our hospice. And Bobby died healed.

Some time ago I told the story of Bobby to a group of nurses, with particular emphasis on Bobby's question in the face of death – 'Has my life been any good?' – my response that I believed it had been good, and the contribution I believed this affirmation of Bobby's worth and value had made in allowing him to finish the business and let go of life. It was clear that one of the nurses was quite agitated by my approach, and in the discussion session she rounded on me with great vehemence. 'How can you call yourself a proper chaplain if you say that this atheist had lived a good life?' she asked. 'How can you say his life had been any good if you do not offer him salvation through Jesus Christ?' I was quite taken aback by the forcefulness of the questions, but I reckoned that they arose from a genuine desire to work out when it was appropriate to share your own faith and when it was not. So we had a person-to-person dialogue for about twenty minutes – while the rest of the participants sat wide-eyed, alternately puzzled and enraptured by the discussion.

I tried to be patient, but it became increasingly clear that far from this young lady's trying to make sense of the appropriateness or otherwise of offering her own faith as a guide and help to her patients, she would be seeking to use it at every opportunity, and would condemn those – hospice chaplain included – who did not do likewise.

Looking back at the exchange of views, it was clearly of value for me to have to think and communicate what I actually believed – though it was not what the young nurse wanted to hear. I remember quoting a verse from the book of Ecclesiastes – at the end of that lovely passage in chapter 3 which tells of the seasons and times of our lives – which reads: 'All we can do is to be happy and do the best we can while we are still alive. All of us should eat and drink and enjoy what we have worked for. It is God's gift.' She didn't think much of that!

Notwithstanding the usefulness of the dialogue, eventually my patience began to wear thin – and it was almost time for a coffee break anyway. So I said, 'Allow me to have the final word. Imagine you are the chaplain, or anyone else on the care team, and Bobby is talking to you. He tells you his life story, he shares with you what he feels he has accomplished by being here, and he asks you, 'Has it been any good? Has my life been worthwhile?' and you say, 'Well, actually, no. You see, you cannot say it's been any good at all unless you give your heart to Jesus,' and he takes a final draw on his roll-up cigarette, and with every last ounce of energy he has he tells you to '**** off!', then the moment of healing is lost, and Bobby will die a restless and embittered man. What do you do then?' 'Oh,' she replied, 'I will go and pray for him.' 'Well,' I responded, 'maybe I should do the same. And, anyway, it's coffee time, and we'll have to stop now in any event.'

At the end of it all, I was exhausted. I went down to our coffee-room to recover. One of the participants from the seminar accompanied me down the stairs. She was on the way to the front door for a smoke. She put her arm round my shoulder and said, 'Heavy stuff, eh?' I grunted in response. 'Never mind,' she continued, 'if it's any consolation, I'm with you.'

At least someone had understood. Bobby had not only taught me the validity of his way of finishing the business, but he had begun to teach other people as well!

So, finishing the business matters. The process for many may not be as dramatic as Bobby's, or as extensive. It may be writing a letter to be left for someone after death comes. It may be saying sorry to a loved one for a hurt caused years ago. It may be seeking absolution from the priest or chaplain for that which stains a life. Or it may be like Andy's process.

Andy, like Bobby, was a retired miner. I liked him a lot, and we had got to know each other very well. One day he looked troubled and I asked him why. 'It's the wife,' he replied. 'Are you worried about how she'll cope?' I asked. 'No, no, she'll cope fine. She's a strong wee woman is my Aggie. No, it's just that I cannae talk wi' her.' 'But you talk together all the time she's in visiting,' I continued. 'Aye, but there's talkin' and there's talkin'. I cannae tell her what I feel. When you've been married as long as we huv, you forget how to say the things that matter.' After a fair exploration of all of this, Andy and I agreed that when his wife came in to visit that afternoon I would stay with them for a bit to see if we could facilitate the "talkin'" Andy needed.

So when Agnes arrived, I told her Andy wanted to speak with her. 'What about?' she asked suspiciously. 'He'll tell you himself,' I replied. 'And he wants me to stay with you both for a while.' 'Why?' she responded, increasingly puzzled. 'You'll see.' Together, we went in to see Andy, propped up on his pillows in a room by himself.

'Here's Agnes,' I began and she sat down and I sat beside Andy on the bed. 'I was telling her you wanted a word.' 'What about?' she said, in an agitated voice. And my heart sank. Had I got it completely wrong? Had I gone too far? 'Tell her what you were telling me this morning,' I continued. 'I was telling you …' he began. 'No, don't tell me again. Tell Agnes.' And with that he turned his head on his pillow towards his wife, smiled a huge smile, and said: 'Och, I luv you, hen.' 'O, Andy, and I love you too.' And she cried, and he cried, and so did their chaplain!

Later that afternoon, Andy and Agnes's daughter came to visit, and Andy was able to share his love with her too. The job had been done. The business had been finished. Healing had happened. It's like that young widower I quoted earlier, now seeing the need to take the time to express the love, to say what needs to be said, to finish the business.

Before I became a hospice chaplain, I had often used at funerals the Scripture verse: 'O death, where is thy victory; O grave, where is thy sting?' simply because it seemed the right thing to say. Now I know it to be true, because of people like Bobby and Andy. At a funeral service I conducted recently, I said of another man, 'He faced death with all that he had, and he won.' That is what Dylan Thomas must have meant when he wrote in one of his poems 'and death shall have no dominion'.

When the business of living is finished, and there is no more that can be done, it is not death but living – in the hands of Bobby and Andy and many more – that has the victory.

Writing your own story

It has been said that everyone has a book in them waiting to be written. I'm not sure about that. But what I do know is that everyone has a story in them waiting to be told. What Bobby was doing was recognising that he had a story worth telling and, though it was a story that he never wrote down, it was worth telling enough to choose someone who would listen as the story unfolded. Bobby chose to do it all at one time. Perhaps if he had done it bit by bit – maybe even before time was running out – or had even tried writing some of it down, he might not have been under so much pressure at the end. So here is an exercise which might be useful.

- Keep a journal for your own private use.

- Or now, with the extensive use of PCs, use a floppy disc to record for your own use what matters to you. (You might already keep a diary or a daily journal. That's fine. But this is slightly different and should be kept separate. It may be that you draw on your diary or personal journal to refresh your memory or help with reflections. Or it may be that you have to start from scratch and have a lot of thinking to do! Either way, the effort will not be wasted.)

- Give the journal a title – your name, or a personal motto, or a quotation that matters to you. Make it unique to you right from the start.

- Look back over significant events or stages of your life.

- Give each one a name – like a chapter heading. This is important, because it anchors each piece of the story and holds it under one heading.

- Write down or record the important parts of that chapter – in headings or in fuller form, whatever works for you. You don't have to be a literary genius. Remember this is an exercise for you and not for wider publication.

- Build the story up bit by bit. It doesn't have to be a continuous record. Add to it when things come up. Slot things in when you remember them. (Which of us can remember things in the right order of events over a long period of time anyway?) Take care and take time.

- Over the months and years, read back over what you have written. Don't change it – that will spoil the spontaneity of your reflections – but add to it and reflect on it in the light of your current situation.

- One day, you may decide to let someone else hear your story. Only you can work out how, with whom and when.

- Above all, enjoy your story. It is unique to you. It matters. And if you ask, like Bobby, 'Has it been any good?' hear a voice saying, 'Yes!' to you now.

A prayer for my dying

I wrote this prayer as part of a workshop during a hospice chaplain's retreat. I found it a very challenging thing to do – and it took me a whole afternoon! I wonder what prayer you might write for your own dying. If you can't or don't wish to write one for yourself, I hope this one may be of help.

God,
accepting of your child,
beyond my understanding or deserving,
let me heed your welcome voice
and know you bid me come.
Embrace me in my dying and your living,
till I find rest in you,
and know my journey is ended,
and I am come home.

Ten

The observation coach

Was none who would be foremost to lead such dire attack;
But those behind cried 'Forward!', and those before cried 'Back!'
Lord Macaulay: Horatius

Let observation with extensive view,
Survey mankind from China to Peru;
Remark each anxious toil, each eager strife,
And watch the busy scenes of crowded life.
Samuel Johnson: The Vanity of Human Wishes

Never having been to either China or Peru, I can make no comment about either country or about the state of humankind in these far-flung corners of the world. I can, however, speak about a country I know well, my own Scotland. And, having spent my childhood under the shadow of Ben Nevis and exploring the beauty of the North West over many years since, I can say from personal observation that one of the most beautiful parts of it is the West Highland Railway Line, and, in particular, the northernmost stretch between the Highland towns of Fort William and Mallaig. And from that railway journey I find an image of 'observation' which can give profound insights into the ways people in the face of death interpret the 'busy scenes of crowded life'.

But first, let me tell you about Nana. Nana – or Maria as she was properly called – was Polish. She had come first to England and then to Scotland at the start of the Second World War, and had lived in a small town in East Lothian. There she had met and then married Vladislav who, like her, had fled Poland and settled in Scotland where he got a job as a miner, a job he had worked at all his working life.

Maria and Vladislav eventually settled in a village just outside Edinburgh where, supported by an extensive Polish community in
Edinburgh and beyond, and bound into the tight miners' community, they brought up a family of three girls, and saw that family
expand into two further generations.

Vladislav had died five years earlier, and Maria had lived on in her
home, supported by her family, until she contracted cancer, became
too ill to live by herself and eventually arrived in our hospice. Her
disease process had thrown up symptoms which we were seeking to
bring under control. Her prognosis was months, and the expectation
was that she would go home after her symptoms had been alleviated,
and only come back to us as and when control of further symptoms
was required.

I got to know all of this from Maria herself, for she was an easy
lady to talk with, and liked nothing better than to engage in long,
rambling conversations, telling me about herself, as well as asking me
about my family life, beliefs, background and lots more. Maria was
one of those open and welcoming people it was a joy to work with.

'Call me Nana,' she once said to me. 'I know it sounds funny, and,
no, I'm not a grandmother to hundreds of children. It's just that
Vladislav called me Nana, and when I hear the name I feel close to
him.' So, Nana it was.

One day when I popped in to see Nana, I saw she had a scrapbook on her knee, a big, floppy scrapbook, most of the pages of
which were already filled with newspaper cuttings, photographs and
pages of typed text. Scattered all over the bed were more of the same,
and, along with them there were two A4 pads which were covered
with closely written script.

'Goodness, Nana!' I exclaimed. 'Blue Peter meets hospice care!'
She smiled, and went on to explain what she was doing. Ever since
her husband had died she had developed a passion to gather information about 'the old days', about her roots in Poland and her early

years of family life in Scotland. So, painstakingly and thoroughly, she had collected what she could – from visits to Poland, from contact with family, from other Polish families, from her own bits and pieces – and was gathering them together in one big scrapbook.

In addition, she was writing down her own reflections, digging deep into her memory for images from childhood, descriptions of her parents and grandparents, memories of war and fear, feelings of separation from homeland and culture, thoughts of her religious up-bringing in the Catholic Church, and much more. She would care-fully write it all down, have it typed up by a friend, revise it further, and have the final copy pasted into the scrapbook as part of her labour of passion and of love.

It was fascinating. She was alive and animated as she told me what she was about, as she shared some of her stories and looked into the past. Over the ensuing months, each time she came into our hospice she would bring the scrapbook and her bag of bits and pieces with her. More work would be done. The scrapbook would be a little fatter, the final story nearer completion.

Whatever the future held for Maria was, to her, largely irrelevant. What would be would be. But for her the important task was look-ing back, seeing where she had come from, reflecting on the journey, and doing so in a clearly tangible fashion.

As we talked, then and on a number of occasions thereafter, the image of a train from Fort William to Mallaig came clearly to mind (I don't know why, but maybe it was because my discussions with her stimulated thoughts of my own childhood). It was an image I shared with Maria, then and later, and one which she clearly understood.

You see, the journey from Fort William to Mallaig on the West Highland line – being the most beautiful in the world! – is very popular with visitors. So, some years ago, to allow the best to be made of the journey, and to permit the maximum enjoyment of the beautiful countryside the train travelled through, the railway company put an observation coach on the back of the train. It was an amazing glass construction – or so it appeared to a small boy when he first saw it – with, as well as big side windows, a glass roof and a glass back to the coach. All of this meant that the passengers could sit in comfort and see where they had come from, see the scenery fall into place behind them, see and reflect on the beauty of the West Highlands in all their glory. Not for them the heeding of the cry 'forward', for that was for someone else to worry about. For them the cry was 'back', to see and to wonder. Not for them the task of driving the train and anticipating what was coming next. Not for them time spent sitting in a regular carriage seeing the scenery flashing by, unable to take it all in. But for them the pleasure of quiet reflection of where they had come from, and seeing everything in its rightful and beautiful place.

For Maria the task was the same. There she sat, looking backwards, seeing the scenes of her life in their proper place, with perspective, with a view of the whole picture. Perhaps for parts of her life she had tried to be up front with the driver. Certainly for many years life had flashed by, too quickly to be appreciated in all its beauty. But now she had time, to reflect, to see where she had come from, to see it all in proper order.

For me – and seeing it clearly illustrated in the task Maria was undertaking – this is both a practical and theological issue. It is practical because it is a necessary part of facing death. Like Bobby and others I have mentioned, it was about 'finishing the business'. For so often people need to see where they have come from, to have someone listen to their story, to be allowed to reflect and see how life has stretched out by seeing where the journey has taken them.

I was once asked to sit with a lady whose husband had died while she was a patient with us and she was too ill to go to the funeral. She and her sister and I got together at the time of her husband's funeral, and after we'd got a cup of tea organised I wasn't too sure what to do next. So I asked her how long she'd been married. 'Fifty-four years,' she replied with pride. And I heard myself continue, 'And I'll bet you can remember your wedding day as if it was yesterday.' 'I can,' she said. 'Do you want to hear about it?' And she told us the whole story, the wedding in the manse because 'big church weddings weren't for the likes of us', the reception – steak pie and peas! – back in her parents' house, a barrel of beer, a fiddler for entertainment. 'Did you have a honeymoon?' I asked. 'No, son, you didnae hae a honeymoon in ma day. Me and ma man had a room in ma sister's hoose, so we went there when the party was o'wer.' 'Well,' I smiled, 'I'll not ask you what you did there!' 'Och, a'll tell you that an a'. I sat on ma man's knee and I stroked his hair. He was a fairmer's laddie and had long hair, bleached blonde wi' the sun. A loved him for his hair. An' I wis seventeen. I kent naithin' aboot whit else to dae. So after a'd stroked his hair for a bit, we went hame tae ma mither's.' And an old lady, at the very moment of her husband's funeral, was wreathed in smiles as she transported herself back to a very special day.

So sitting in the observation car and looking backwards can be supremely useful and important, as a dying person makes sense of where they have come from and what it all means.

But this is also a theological issue. Which of us knows what the future holds? Yet do we not seek to enter into the will and mind of God to see and know, or even to direct and influence, what the next stage of the journey might contain? Disturbed by how life flashes by as we look out of the carriage window, do we not try to work our way up to the engine to get some control, to look for an under-standing of our destiny? Do we not often use prayer like that, even to seek to impose our will on the mind of God so that the direction we take is of our choosing, our desire being to have a God who is responsive to our whim?

If this is our approach – and, for me at least, it is an approach which I fall into again and again even despite myself – perhaps the task, our need in communion with God and in reflective prayer, is to sit in the observation car at the rear of the train. There, we can see where we have come from, see this and that fall into its proper place, find a perspective, and believe and know that if our God has guided us thus far, we can trust him enough to take us on to the next stage.

On her final admission to us, Maria had no scrapbook and bag of bits and pieces with her. 'No work to do, Nana?' I asked her. She smiled, and replied, 'No more work to do. My story is told.' The following day, surrounded by her family, Nana died peacefully.

People often ask me, 'Why did you go into ministry? Did you feel a call? Was there writing on the wall?' And I have to say that my answer is often along the lines of 'Well, I don't really know.' It's not that I have never felt called, or sure in my mind that I was being about God's business. But I can really only discern that with clarity by looking backwards, seeing how thing are in their proper place – influences, guidance, events, problems, failures, successes, decisions, and all the rest.

I don't know what God will have me do tomorrow. I don't know what direction he will have me take. But I trust that if what I see behind me today makes sense, and has taken me thus far, then I can trust that when I look back tomorrow, what I have experienced today will also make sense as part of the journey of God's purpose for my life.

I did not understand

I did not understand
the why
and the how
of this suffering-time.
Could it not pass?
Would it always be like this,
for ever,
blotting out all else?
And why?
What purpose did it serve?
And was this God's doing,
this cruel God
to make me suffer this?
I did not understand.
I did not wish to understand,
just to be rid of this moment,
this all-consuming moment
of pain.

Look, now,
there it is
that moment of pain.
Look now,
it's part of what you are.
Look, now,
and see it
in the one great panorama
of living.

Look, now.
Don't be troubled now about understanding.

Just look,
and know.

I did not want to remember.
For remembering is to relive,
and to relive is to cry again.
The photograph told me I should remember,
so it lies face down in the drawer.
The poppy called me to remember,
so I did not watch or share in Remembrance.
The smell,
the scene,
the dress,
the ring,
all prompted me to remember,
and all brought back the tears.
So why remember?
Why go back
and go through it again?
Why cry
when crying brings
only the emptiness that is to be filled
with more remembering?
I did not want to remember
if it would always be like this.

Look, now,
and remember again.
No, do not dry your tears
for they are part of your looking.
Look, now,

and see it all.
And see what sits beside your remembering
and makes you smile.

I did not want to forget,
leaving behind what I only experienced
for so short a time,
the colour and the sound
that lifted me on wings of pleasure,
the smile,
the tender touch,
the warm embrace
that made me live.
I did not want to forget
how feelings made me
rise above my ordinary living.
I did not want to forget.

Will the scene fade,
and leave me with a yearning
for what has been so rich
but is now no more?
Will life give me pleasure
and then not allow me to cherish
for longer than a moment?
I did not want to forget.

Look, now,
and know that forgetting is impossible.
It's there,
and there,
and there,
that which you feared you'd lost.
Look, now,

and gaze again upon that moment
and know it matters still.

I did not want to let go
that moment of joy.
It was as if everything that had ever been
had prepared me for that instant.
I did not want to let go,
but, instead, to stay
and shelter in the rapture of all that was good
and right
and true.
But,
I had to leave behind that which gave me that all-important glimpse
of life in all its fullness.
So I moved on,
wondering why the joy was so fleeting,
pondering whether I'd ever experienced it at all,
when I struggled with pain and loss.

Look, now,
for even time cannot force you to let go.
Look, now,
and look again.
You did not carelessly abandon
this that was your moment.
Look, now,
and live again.

Look, now,
and learn
that life in all its fullness
has been yours.

My God, I tried

My God, I tried to know and understand
your ways and your direction,
yet could not see or grasp the how and where,
the why and when and what of this too hectic journey.

My God, I tried to watch it all go by,
to take it in and know that all was well.
But life was fast and stops were few
and this mere mind could not absorb it all.

My God, I tried to look behind and see it all unfold,
and now I know that all that's been is there
to take me here and point the way ahead,
the way I did not know.

My God, I tried too hard to be in charge,
to take control and know the way I had to go
and how to get there on my own.
But now I know it is not me but you who takes me on,
and shows me now that all is well
the journey through.

Eleven

Damming the stream

Even the weariest river winds somewhere safe to sea.
Algernon Charles Swinburne: The Garden of Proserpine

By the rivers of Babylon we sat down;
there we wept when we remembered Zion.
Psalm 137:1

Some years before I took the decision to leave the parish ministry and enter hospice chaplaincy, I attended a day course specifically designed for 'ministers in mid-ministry'. It was a good day, exploring with others at the same stage of ministry as myself, looking at how we had coped with the years of service we had given to the Church, and sharing how we saw things developing for us in the future.

As part of the day we were given an exercise to do on our own: to draw or paint or sketch a river, symbolising the journey of ministry we had experienced thus far, and how we saw it flowing into the future. It was a thought-provoking exercise, and for me a very challenging and enlightening one – particularly because I had to represent my thoughts in artistic form and not in the words which have always been my stock-in-trade. The nature of my river, what it meant to me at the time and the clarity it began to give me about my future were very revealing, and a great help in focusing my thinking about my ministry. The interpretation of it is, perhaps, the subject of another book! But the image of the river, and its usefulness in my present work, has never left me.

And it is an image, in a quite specific form, which I have begun to use with people who are struggling to cope with bereavement.

I referred in an earlier chapter to the patient who felt he had lost his 'connectedness' in the face of the knowledge that he was going to die. This loss of purpose, of a sense that the stages of life are linked, is experienced equally deeply in the process of grief following a death. Or, to turn it round the other way, the sense that there is no understanding of what the next stage will be, the separation of the future from all that the past has contained, is a devastating emotion for bereaved people. 'I cannot think of life without him'; 'How can I face the future alone?'; 'She was my everything' and a host of similar statements and questions indicate very strongly that bereaved people find it almost impossible to conceptualise a future without the ongoing presence of the person who has died.

The turmoil and turbulence of grief are so shattering to the individual because the very beliefs, attitudes and sense of continuity that give life meaning have been profoundly challenged. Grief is so devastating because it feels as though the rules of living have suddenly been changed.

It is almost impossible – or should I say, it is completely impossible – for anyone who has not experienced the devastation of the death of a loved one to understand these feelings of turmoil, this sudden changing of the rules. This is particularly true in dealing with someone who has lost a partner. Even for myself, dealing with the death of parents, relatives and friends gives me scant insight into the loss of a spouse. I instance two expressions of my own lack of understanding.

I remember in my early years of ministry visiting a Christian lady whose husband had recently died. They had been married for over fifty years, and had both lived exemplary Christian lives. She was inconsolable in her grief when I visited her after the funeral. In my short ministry up to that point I had never seen such intensity of loss. So in my 'sensitivity' as a Christian minister I suggested to her that death for a Christian was a joy of being able to claim a promised place in God's eternal Kingdom and that one day she and her husband would be reunited in the nearer presence of God. The old lady lifted her head from her hands and gave me what I can only describe as a withering stare! Her face said it all: 'You do not understand. Of course I believe what you say, but that is irrelevant to me at this time. Just allow me to be broken, because that is how I feel.'

Some years later as I stood in the grounds of a hospice and cried inconsolably at the death of a young friend, and cursed God for his unfairness, I understood for the first time what that lady had been through.

I also recall my work with a young woman before and after the death of her husband. She had been left with three young children. Her beautiful love, marriage and husband were all gone. She talked about suicide. She made it clear that life wasn't worth living. She told me how she would go to her husband's grave and cry out that she wanted to be with him because life without him was so totally empty. I remember thinking that she had her three children, that she was young and vibrant, that she could even get married again. Thank God I had picked up enough sense along the way to stop myself from verbalising such insensitive platitudes! But still I simply did not understand how empty and alone she felt, and had no insight into her desire to end it all.

It is working with these issues, and trying to understand the depth of feelings in these situations of loss, that takes me back to the picture of the river. It is a picture which is still evolving, but which, when shared with bereaved people as a way of helping understand their loss, seems to make sense.

Life is a stream, like a burn tumbling through highland heather and bracken, flowing along with its twists and turns, rapids and calmer parts, sometimes taking an unexpected turn, sometimes flowing predictably onwards. Then, suddenly, a huge boulder comes careering down the hillside and falls smack, bang in the middle of the stream. It is big and heavy, and it completely blocks the flow of the water. So, for the moment, in the devastation of that natural phenomenon, the stream dies. There is no flow beyond the boulder. All that is left is a waterless bed, exposed, lifeless, useless.

It is the suddenness and totality of death which makes the image of the devastation wrought by the boulder so real. I have lost count of the number of times when, even in the hospice setting people are taken completely by surprise when the moment of death comes – despite all the preparation there has been: talking, finishing the business, anticipating and, sometimes, praying for it to happen when it is taking too long. It is as if the 'where there is life there is hope' feeling has contrived to block out the knowledge that 'in the midst of life we are in death'. The devastation of the death is all too apparent. The damming of the stream is as complete as it is sudden. The meaning of life is gone. The damage of the boulder is total.

I remember walking to the front door of our hospice with Alice, a grieving widow, following the death of her husband. She now had to face making funeral arrangements and all the pain that this entailed. She stopped at the door and began to rummage in her handbag. She took out a cheque book and opened it. I thought she was going to give us a donation! But far from writing a cheque, she began to cry. 'Jim gave me this last week and he said "You'll have to deal with this now, Alice." And now that I've got it I don't know what to do. I've never even written a cheque before. Jim always saw to things like that.' For this broken woman, facing the future with all its uncertainties and aloneness, with its implications of dealing with business affairs and bills and paperwork, was quite overwhelming. Of course there were people who could help her, but they weren't Jim. At that moment, and symbolised by an unused cheque book, the future was too frightening to comprehend.

It is no use saying that Alice and Jim should have prepared themselves for this, or lived a more 'modern marriage' with more sharing of responsibilities. Who prepares themselves totally for this sense of devastation, this aloneness? And who can? The reality was that at that moment the boulder of the death of Alice's life-partner had cut off any meaningful future. It had done its terrible job. The stream of meaningful life had been dammed.

Every time a bereaved person looks for the familiar interactions to turn life back to how it was and this does not occur, the reality and the finality of the loss are reinforced. So bereaved people like Alice feel that survival is impossible without the deceased, and that the pain is too great to be tolerated.

So, with the picture of the boulder damming the stream I have begun to appreciate why bereaved people feel that survival is impossible, and to understand them when they say, 'Life's not worth living any more.'

Some time after Jim died, I recall Alice telling me how she felt. 'When Jim died – and, I suppose, when someone of major importance in anyone's life dies – it is as if the world you have known and become familiar with has stopped, though life somehow still seems to be going on all around you. The phone rings, there's shopping to do, meals to prepare, a house to tidy. And the people around you are going about their daily business. And there you sit in the middle of it all, starting a letter, or trying to concentrate on forms from the Inland Revenue or instructions from the solicitor, and talk about widow's benefit and funeral arrangements and arranging for wreaths to be chosen. You might respond to a question. Your hands move. But your heart's not in it. The real me was somehow standing at the edge of the room, watching, wondering, "How does she do it? How does she function?" For me, I felt I was walking through treacle.'

What does it feel like for you to have this boulder completely block your stream, to feel that your known world has stopped? Only a bereaved person who has lost someone of major importance in their life can tell you.

The image, however, does not stop there. In our ongoing work with bereaved families and individuals, the process of grief is worked upon and affirmed. People come to check out the unfolding of their lives, week by week, month by month, stage by stage. They come because they need to be listened to; to hear that their strange and new feelings are a normal part of the process; to find reassurance that the periods of regression, moments of deep sadness which hit them in waves at times they least expect them, do not mean that they are cracking up or being depressed or behaving abnormally; to talk about their loved one when few people are prepared to listen any more. And it is in this continuation of the grief process that I find I am developing the image of the river in a number of other ways.

I am no geophysicist, but I know that water has an insidious habit of finding its way past obstacles. Slowly it can erode stone, destroy river banks, find a passage through cracks and fissures. Water will find its way. A stream will not be blocked for ever. So it is with this great boulder which has dammed the stream. The water building up behind it will, bit by bit, day by day, find a path round the boulder. It will take time. It may be hidden for a long while. But it will happen and, on one side or another of the great boulder, a trickle of water will appear again.

The process of bereavement is like that. Of course there is the feeling that once the river has been dammed there is no future for the flow of the stream. But it is the task of those of us who work with bereaved people to wait with them, to listen to them, to affirm them in their devastation, and to point out the little trickles of water that begin to flow round the boulder. It is our task to help bereaved people to see the stream beginning to move again.

Shirley's mother had been with us for a number of weeks through a long course of palliative chemotherapy. It was clear that Shirley and her mother were devoted to each other. A widowed mother, an only daughter, two caring and loving people, and a great deal of support and understanding. All that needed to be said had been said. The business had been finished. Shirley was well prepared for her mother's death. Her mother was prepared to go. The hospice setting had accommodated the needs of both of them very well.

What Shirley was not prepared for was the devastation she felt when her mother died – not instantly, but shortly afterwards. During the first few weeks the funeral, the clearing of a house, the reflection on the process of dying all served to 'keep Shirley going'. Her faith was exemplary, her church very supportive. Shirley had done well. She was handling her grief as admirably as she had handled the dying process.

A month after the death it all fell apart. She found herself unable to control her tears. She couldn't sleep. People had told her she was a remarkable woman, an example to others. She felt so herself. So what was happening? What had gone wrong? And would it ever be right again?

The first thing we did with Shirley was to help her see that what she was experiencing was normal. The devastation of grief takes many forms, and none of them is extraordinary of itself. Then, slowly, month by month in our meetings for relatives, we accompanied Shirley on her journey. We worked through birthdays, Christmas, New Year and the like. We heard how on occasions when she least expected it she had broken down in tears – at the January sales, when an old black-and-white movie came on the TV, when 'Songs of Praise' chose her favourite hymn. But slowly and steadily she moved on. We were able to talk of the normality of what she was going through, but also to help her see how things were changing, improving, moving.

We worked with Shirley up to the anniversary of her mother's death. She coped with that much better than she had expected. Now we only see her from time to time. She tells me of the odd bad day, but also of changes and developments in her life. She tells me of talking with her mother, of closeness, of warmth. She tells me of her engagement and her new job. She tells me of a stream that is flowing again.

It is clear, therefore, that once the stream begins to flow on the other side of the boulder, it will not take the path of the stream when it flowed before. It may have been dammed up for so long that it has to take a different course. The boulder has blocked the stream right enough. But it has also changed the direction of the flow.

Life after a death will be different. It is hard to contemplate. Indeed, it is the prospect of its being radically different that makes people scared for that future. C.S. Lewis wrote: 'No one ever told me that grief felt so much like fear.'

It is fear of the unknown, fear of change, fear of life's direction being radically different that makes the prospect of facing what lies on the other side of the boulder impossible to comprehend. Bereaved people need gentle affirmation and guidance not only to see the trickle of water beginning to flow again, but to see that the change of direction of the stream can be renewing and enlivening and full of possibilities and growth.

The final use of the image of the stream comes in this way. I think the worst thing that can be said to the bereaved at any stage is something like, 'You'll get over it.' I remember Shirley saying, five months after her mother had died, 'The worst thing is that they [her family] don't talk about Mum any more. They avoid it like the plague. It's as if she didn't exist. It's as if she didn't matter any more. It's as if she'd never existed.'

Bereaved people don't want to be told that they will get over a death, because it will sound dismissive both of their own feelings and, as this young lady made clear, of the person they need to remember. So, going back to our image of the stream, it is obvious that the boulder remains where it has fallen, damming the stream and stopping the flow. The water has found its way and the stream has slowly begun to flow again. The course of the stream has now changed and the flow is different from anything which could have been contemplated before the boulder did its worst. But the boulder remains, as a permanent symbol of this dramatic event, this cataclysmic change which the loss has created. The death will never to be 'got over', but is a fixed point at which the river of life altered its course.

Each one of us has to journey through life holding in our being two important truths – if we love, we are opening a door to riches beyond imagining, and yet when we do so we open ourselves to the pain and agony of loss. So, what are we to do? Are we not to love for fear of the pain of loss? Or are to we to find the riches of love and recognise and work through losses which may ensue?

If we love, we will know the pain of loss. Nothing is more certain. And that loss will devastate us, it will change us and it will renew us. To deal with it requires time, patience, assurance, wisdom, insight and compassion. The key, then, is surely to help bereaved people to learn to bear the pain of loss that must inevitably be faced, and to show that the river can flow again, and that there can be life on the other side.

The key issue for me is to help bereaved people to see the signs of new beginnings, and to celebrate the flowing on of the stream into growth and newness and fullness of life again.

Perhaps that is why I don't get depressed working with bereaved people. I would even say that I enjoy it, and it is among the most rewarding parts of my work. It is a genuine privilege to wait and watch, to listen and share, and see life begin again when those who have been bereaved would never have thought it possible.

Just a trickle
(A meditation on Ezekiel chapter 47)

The man led me back to the entrance of the Temple. Water was coming out from under the entrance and flowing east, the direction the Temple faced. It was flowing down from under the south side of the Temple past the south side of the altar. The man then took me out of the temple area by way of the north gate and led me round to the gate that faces east. A small stream of water was flowing out at the south side of the gate. With his measuring-rod the man measured five hundred metres downstream to the east and told me to wade through the stream there. The water came only to my ankles. Then he measured another five hundred metres, and the water came up to my knees. Another five hundred metres further down, the water was up to my waist. He measured five hundred more, and there the stream was so deep I could not wade through it. It was too deep to cross except by swimming. He said to me, 'Mortal man, note all this carefully.' Then the man took me to the bank of the river, and when I got there I saw that there were very many trees on each bank. He said to me, '... Wherever the stream flows, there will be all kinds of animals and fish. The stream will make the water of the Dead Sea fresh, and wherever it flows it will bring life ... There will be fishermen on the shore of the sea, and they will spread out their nets there to dry. There will be as many different kinds of fish there as there are in the Mediterranean sea ... On each bank of the stream all kinds of trees will grow to provide food. Their leaves will never wither, and they will never stop bearing fruit. They will have fresh fruit every month, because they are watered by the stream which flows from the Temple, and their leaves will be used for healing people.'

'It's just a trickle of water,' I said to the man,
just a trickle,
running from under the door,
along the terrace.
'What good is that?' I said to the man.
'What's that tell me?
There's a tap running?
There's a burst pipe?
There's a leaking cistern?
I told you this place was a mess,
this Temple,
a useless monolith from which nothing good could come.
It's just a trickle of water,' I said to the man.
'What good is that?'

And the man said, 'Walk in the water
for as long as I will measure.'

'So, I'm walking in the water,' I murmured to the man.
'Wet feet, a gentle paddle, like a stroll by the seaside.
So?
I'm doing it now, just as you said.
Why?
I don't know.
I'm walking in the water,' I murmured to the man.
'What good is that?'

And the man said, 'Walk in the water
for as long as I will measure.'

'Now, I'm wading in the water,' I called to the man.
'And getting very wet indeed!
It's been a while now and I'm still going on.

I think I'd prefer to be back on the terrace –
you know, when it was just a trickle?
I'm not sure I like this much.
I'm wading in the water,' I called to the man.
'What good is that?'

And the man said, 'Walk in the water
for as long as I will measure.'

'Good God, I'm treading water,' I cried to the man.
'Treading water, right here in the middle of this stream.
Stream? Where did this stream come from?
What happened to the trickle,
the gentle paddle,
my feet still touching the bottom?
I don't like treading water.
The current, the depth, the flow …
Help me! I'm treading water!' I cried to the man.
'What good is that?'

And the man said, 'There's the bank, then.
Head for shore – and rest a while.'

'So, I'm resting by the water,' I gasped to the man.
'I'm resting, all right.
But what now?
What good was that …?

'Wow!
Where's this?
I thought it was desert down here –
at least that's what I'd been told.
But look at all of this.
Did you know there were trees out here, and flowers –
goodness, look at the flowers,
and the fruit on the trees,
and the animals,
and the birds …
I thought nothing lived out here.
People told me nothing could survive in this wilderness.
Now here I am – and it's amazing!
And – yes – there are folk over there –
fishing from the bank …
Any luck, chaps?
Maybe I'll come and join you!

'So, I'm resting by the water,' I gasped to the man.
'Why did you not tell me it was going to be like this?'

And the man said, 'There's the stream,
all the way back from where you started.
Look, way back there – look – and wonder …'

'So, I'm looking at the water,' I said to the man.
'I'm looking … back there …
Well, now! Isn't that something?
The water came from …
the monolith,

the temple,
that big,
useless,
immovable obstacle
to progress and movement …
The water … came from … there …
The trickle … has created this?
And I've gone with the flow?
So, I'm looking at the water,' I said to the man,
'I'm looking back there …
and I am absolutely amazed!'

And the man said, 'In a while, sometime soon,
I'll show you another trickle of water,
another beginning of another stream.
Not yet, but when you're ready to move on –
even when you're not sure you're ready to move on –
In a while I'll show you …
I'll tell you – to walk in the water
for as long as I will measure.'

Reflecting on how you move on after a trauma

The two fundamental problems faced by people who are bereaved are an overwhelming sense of loneliness (Who can you really tell what is happening to you?) and a worry about what is normal in grief (When so much you are dealing with is new and strange, how do you know what is appropriate or out of the ordinary?).

Sometimes there may be a self-help group you can be part of, where people who themselves have been or are going through bereavement can listen, give reassurance and show they understand. Or it may be a trusted friend who can tell you that you're not going mad, and that what you are feeling is OK. Or it may be your GP or counsellor or pastor who will give you the reassurance you need. (And remember, the need for that reassurance and the willingness to give it has to go on for a lot longer than our present society deems it necessary.)

But often people who are bereaved have no group or individual to whom they can turn, and, even if they do, they don't want to bother people over and over again with the same stuff that has been shared before. It is then that the loneliness and confusion can often be overwhelming.

If you are in that position, here is an exercise, based on the picture in this past chapter, which may be of benefit – in two ways: to help you to be honest with yourself about what you feel at different stages of the grief process, and to help you see signs of moving on, which we sometimes miss because we are living day by day so close to our sorrow.

- Find for yourself a notebook, big enough that you can see clearly what is written and drawn on the pages. Keep it safe and away from prying eyes. This is for you and no one else to see!

- Draw yourself a stream. Don't worry about how it looks. It's your picture, and so it's already good. And, anyway, no one else is going to see it!

- Write alongside it the stages that matter to you, the twists and turns, the rapids and smooth stretches along the way.

- As the stream flows on, write down what you planned for, where you hoped the stream would take you, your expectations, dreams and prayers.

- You may not have enough space, for the past, present and future, on your picture. So on a separate page, write down what has mattered to you in past stages, what life is like in the present, and what you had looked forward to in days to come.

- Take time over this. Go back to it. Change it and adapt it. Only you know what should be there.

- Then put a boulder in the stream.

- Write down the effects of that huge and devastating event.

- Be angry. Be devastated. Be confused. Be whatever you need to be. And, above all, be honest.

- Write, somewhere, what of the future is now gone. Take your list of hopes and dreams and promises and find out what is no longer possible – and why. Write down your feelings about your losses – remembering that one boulder brings lots of losses.

- You might wish to draw your stream again – seeing clearly what should have been there and isn't now because of the damage the boulder has caused.

- And leave it there for now. That is enough for a while, as you get in touch with the effects of loss.

- One day, take your notebook, turn to a fresh page, and write TRICKLES in big letters at the top. Each time something good happens, some achievement, some success, some 'doing it for the first time', or whatever, write it down. If it happens again, write it down again.

- If something bad happens, go back and write it against the dried-up bed of your stream. But always remember to write on the 'trickles' page, no matter how small the trickles might seem to be. You are going to need that page – or even pages – for a long time.

- Some day, draw a picture of a stream again – maybe even superimposed on the old one – and see the new direction the trickles have created for the stream. See that it is flowing again.

- Write down once more your hopes and plans and dreams for the future. Take time to revisit the boulder too, and see how, trickle by insignificant trickle, you have moved on.

Twelve

The growing child

I would not coddle the child.
Samuel Johnson, from Boswell's Life of Johnson

When I was a child, my speech, feelings, and thinking were all those of a child; now that I am a man, I have no more use for childish ways.
I Corinthians 13:11

Of all the people I have worked with in the bereavement process, Cathie's grief seemed to be the deepest. Cathie was a 55-year-old woman, divorced in her early twenties after a short and disastrous marriage, and whose aunt, Susan, had been a patient with us for a number of weeks. Susan was a lovely lady, just ten years older than her niece, and the two of them had lived together since Cathie was 13, Cathie only leaving home for the couple of years of her marriage and returning when it all fell apart. Cathie's mother had died, and she had never known her father. Susan and her husband had taken her into their home, and she became their family. They had no children of their own, and when Susan's husband was killed in a mining accident shortly after Cathie's return home, Cathie and Susan became almost inseparable. It is easy enough to see how in their losses, one by divorce and the other by death, these two women had found solace and support in each other. They were more like sisters than aunt and niece. And the gentle and quiet Cathie was cared for and protected by the stronger and bolder Susan.

So it remained until Susan was diagnosed as having liver cancer. During her three weeks in our hospice she and I talked a great deal about her concerns for Cathie. Understandably, she was fearful as to how Cathie would cope. I reassured her that we and others would look out for this vulnerable woman and do our best to help. When Susan died, I conducted her funeral. Cathie was devastated, as broken by a death as anyone I have seen in twenty-five years of ministry.

Not surprisingly, in the days and weeks following, many people began to express their concern for Cathie. Neighbours, her GP, our own staff – myself included – all feared for her ability to cope. And so, even before Cathie began to be involved with our bereavement after-care service, I arranged for her to come to see me.

This frail, quiet-spoken, frightened woman was indeed devastated by grief. She wept openly. She talked about having nothing to live for. She said that she had lost an aunt, a friend, a sister, a companion, a confidante, a mainstay, and much more, all at the one time. She wanted to die, to end her life, simply to be reunited with Susan. It was heart-rending to listen to.

I myself, the GP, another member of our staff, and those of us who are involved with bereavement after-care in our hospice worked with Cathie for a long while. We listened, journeyed with her, encouraged, empathised, week by week, month by month. As well as attending our support meetings, Cathie met with me regularly, and there were times, to be honest, when I wondered how things would turn out and whether I had the ability to work with her any further or to offer her any constructive help. I'm still working with Cathie. At the time of writing this there are signs of progress. But it is very, very slow, and the process of adapting to the loss of her aunt is taking a long time.

There seemed to be something missing in my understanding of the depth of her grief, the slowness of her adjustment and the struggle to cope. It was something to do with C.S. Lewis's observation about grief being like fear. Cathie looked and sounded frightened. It was as if she did not want to cope. It was as if it was all too much, not worth the bother of trying. More than once she talked of suicide. So for my sake if not for hers I needed an image, a picture which would help me understand her situation, and help me get a grip on my own feelings.

One day when she had come to see me and was telling me what the past few days had held for her, I looked across at this frail soul, and the picture came to me. Let me explain.

I have three children, the eldest of whom went to university in 1994. She had a place in the Law Faculty of Aberdeen University and, on the appointed day, she and I drove to Aberdeen from Edinburgh for Fresher's week and her moving into halls of residence. For the whole family it was a mixture of excitement and apprehension, and that's how my daughter and I felt as we unloaded her stuff and got things organised in her room in halls.

Eventually it came time for me to leave to drive back home. We said our farewells, gave each other a big hug, and I got in the car and drove out of the halls' car-park. I waved from the car window, and as I looked back I saw this very young lass, slim, frail, no more than a child, standing on the steps and waving goodbye. She looked so vulnerable, so alone, so unready for this great adventure of university life. I knew she'd cope. She knew she'd cope. But the picture of a young woman alone on the steps is etched on my mind for ever.

And it was this picture of the child in a big, new, exciting but frightening world that I saw as I looked across at Cathie – a child growing up and launching out on her own. It was as if she was having to be an adult for the first time, and face the big world by herself – having been protected and nurtured for so many years by a loving Susan.

So often the pain and emptiness a bereaved person feels is about anxiety and helplessness. Psychologists will confirm that these aspects of loss are a product of what has affected us profoundly in childhood, early experiences of separation and the associated anxieties. So it is in this pain of separation that those who are bereaved seek the comfort and consolation of others. Yet what consolation can be offered, when all the bereaved person craves for, cries out for, is the return of the dead person? For life has no meaning, deep feelings of fear and anxiety cannot be dispelled, unless that happens.

What Cathie wanted, what she needed most, was for someone to say that Susan was still there, that there was a haven of refuge to which she could return when the big, frightening world became too overwhelming for her. She needed that reassurance which my daughter has always had that there was a home to return to, a place of security and rest and support, in which to be restored and renewed, and from which to launch out again to cope with the wide world.

Now that Susan was dead, Cathie had no such place, no such security. She had been left as a vulnerable child on the steps of this big world, and she was alone and very scared.

Such is the overwhelming need to have the dead person back that often a bereaved person may even seek to push away the help and compassion that is offered by others. For Cathie, the passion was to have Susan back, to hold her from the finality of death. And as with other bereaved people in Cathie's situation, all other relationships seemed to fade in comparison with this intense focus and longing. Not surprisingly, therefore, as others will surely experience, at times I felt cut off by this bereaved woman, rejected, unwanted and frequently quite impotent to help, when the one who had gone was wanted so much.

To be honest, this feeling of being pushed away brought with it a sense of despair for me, and a deep examination of whether I was doing anything useful at all with Cathie, and even a questioning of my own abilities. So it was the image of the vulnerable child, seemingly abandoned to the world, that not only helped me understand how Cathie felt, but began to help me understand my own feelings of helplessness in dealing with her.

I spoke recently with a woman whose mother was dying. Her father had died when she was four years old, and her mother had been her sole carer for over fifty years. The closeness of her mother's death brought with it not only the loss of the most important person in her life, but the prospect of being an orphan, of having no parents at all. 'I don't think I'm ready to be an "oldie",' she told me. 'I don't think I want to be the "senior generation" when my mother dies. I don't know if I'm prepared for this responsibility.'

So it is not just little children who become orphaned. We can become an orphan at any age, from childhood to the 'senior generation'. And whatever our age, we have to face the devastating fact that we have no parents at all.

What does this mean for us? It means that there is no one who will care for us for no other reason than that we are their child. There is no one automatically responsible for us. But there's more. For the other side of the coin is that there is also no one to give us a hard time because they are always our parent, and no one for whom we have to feel responsible when they reach old age and infirmity. That which is 'mutual' between us – duties, obligations, relationships, history, responsibilities – has ended, gone for ever. In a very real sense, the death of both parents completes our childhood, whether we are still technically a child or assumed to be an adult. In so doing, it brings an end to a significant part of our lives.

For Cathie, Susan's death forced her to complete her childhood even though she was an adult. It was this sudden facing of adulthood that made Cathie very scared.

It remains our ongoing task, therefore, to help Cathie and others like her to be adults in an adult world. It will not be easy in Cathie's case, and is all the more difficult because in her relationship with Susan there was little or no preparation for this period of her life. But we believe we can make it. We believe that Cathie can stand on her own feet. And we will go on helping her with that.

Before I leave this issue, let me offer the following thought. I began this chapter by saying that Cathie's grief at the loss of her aunt was as intense as I have ever known. The picture of the vulnerable child and my reflections on how I can work with this at least help me understand the depth of Cathie's grief and my own reactions to it. But it also gives me a clue to this business about the death of our parents, even though the deaths of each of them may be some years apart. It is an image, therefore, which I can and do make my own.

As I write this, my own mother has been dead for over twenty years and my father died a couple of years ago at the age of eighty-two. My sister and I are now the oldest generation left in our immediate family line. When my father died I remembered the image I had used with Cathie. I felt myself to be standing as a child on the steps of a hall of residence feeling the vulnerability of being alone in a big world. I hoped I would cope, and that in some fashion, at least, I was ready for that moment. So working with Cathie helped me to begin see the picture a little more clearly, and from her I have learned a little better how to face my own bereavement process.

When I was a child
(A reflection on part of 1 Corinthians 13)

I may be able to speak the languages of men and even of angels, but if I have no love, my speech is no more than a noisy gong or a clanging cymbal. I may have the gift of inspired preaching; I may have all knowledge and understand all secrets; I may have all the faith needed to move mountains – but if I have no love, I am nothing. I may give away everything I have, and even give my body to be burnt – but if I have no love, this does me no good. Love is patient and kind; it is not jealous or conceited or proud; love is not ill-mannered or selfish or irritable; love does not keep a record of wrongs; love is not happy with evil, but is happy with the truth. Love never gives up; and its faith, hope, and patience never fail. Love is eternal. There are inspired messages, but they are temporary; there are gifts of speaking in strange tongues, but they will cease; there is knowledge, but it will pass. For our gifts of knowledge and of inspired messages are only partial; but when what is perfect comes, then what is partial will disappear. When I was a child, my speech, feelings, and thinking were all those of a child; now that I am a man, I have no more use for childish ways. What we see now is like a dim image in a mirror; but then we shall see face to face. What I know now is only partial; then it will be complete – as complete as God's knowledge of me. Meanwhile these three remain: faith, hope and love; and the greatest of these is love.

When I was a child
I played,
and in my playing
found a world where I belonged.

Now that I'm grown,
help me to find that belonging again,
so that,
being finished with childish things,
I do not lose the me that is really me.

When I was a child
I cried,
and in my crying found comfort
in a warm breast
and a full embrace.

Now that I'm grown,
help me to cry again,
and know that I am yet enfolded to the breast
of a Love that understands.

When was a child
I screamed
and in my fear
found a presence that would banish
the darkness of my troubled soul.

Now that I'm grown,
help me not to stifle the scream,
believing again in that Presence
which even now conquers
my evil night.

When I was a child
I believed
that all was simple
and easy to understand.
Now that I'm grown
help me to dig into the uncertainties
and find again that which I know
to be clear
and right
and true.

When I was a child
I knew,
with absolute certainty,
that love mattered.

Now that I'm grown,
help me to know
as I am known,
to love
as I am loved,
and to know Love as Love should be known.

When I was a child
I slept,

with untroubled ease,
the gentle sleep of peaceful dreams.

Now that I'm grown,
give me that rest,
that I may sleep
and dream untroubled
of gentle peace.

When I was a child,
I awoke,
to the unbounded excitement
of a new day.

Now that I'm grown,
make me excited again
with the promise of new beginnings
and a day fresh with possibilities.

When I was a child
things lasted for ever,
and the moment of joy
was all that mattered.

Now that I'm grown,
there are other moments
to overwhelm the moment of joy.
So tell me again what lasts for ever –
about faith,
hope,
and love,
that I am not overwhelmed any more.

For all my days

When I was young, you nurtured me,
fed me and clothed me, held me and loved me,
and let me learn and grow and find my way.
When I questioned and challenged
you listened, corrected me and guided me,
rebuked me and affirmed me,
and helped me know and understand and love what I am.
When I left you, you watched me,
you did not stop or hold me,
or restrain me or revile me,
you let me go, believing in me and my going.
When I missed you, I cried at my leaving you,
at my frailty in coping without you,
your security and warmth, your healing and strength.
When I missed you I missed you more than I can say.
Now, when I remember you,
in your nurture and purpose for me,
and your healing and sustaining of me,
in your strength and commitment to me,
there is no leaving now,
no separating, no going, no returning,
only being in you and with you
for all my days.

Thirteen

The damaged painting

Paint my picture truly like me, all these roughnesses, pimples, warts and everything as you see it.
Oliver Cromwell, from Walpole's Anecdotes of Painting

Tell me what's happening in your picture.
A father to a child

Hanging on the wall of my office is a painting, not of any scene in particular, but of an imaginary place: a country church, a barn and a little white cottage by a bend in a river, surrounded by trees and hills and with a very atmospheric sky. My wife and I bought it together some years ago simply because we liked it, and it hung for a while in the sitting room of our home.

When we moved to a smaller house, we had no room for such a large painting, so we decided that it would be best in my office. But when I was moving my bits and pieces, the painting got bumped against the corner of a table and was damaged – not badly, but enough to put a mark on the picture. It's not a big mark, but it is one that can't be removed as the paint has been scored.

To be honest, I was frightened to tell my wife, fearful of her reaction. Such a lovely picture had been spoiled, and although I am still attached to it, and it still hangs in my office, there is now a permanent flaw in something otherwise perfect.

Some years ago Rita came to see me in my office. Rita was a widow, and had been married for over forty years. Her husband, Stan, had died at home in the loving care of his wife and family. At the end, death was a blessed release, and he had died with dignity and at peace. Rita herself was a most dignified lady and, in the process of sharing in her grief, it became clear that she was at peace with herself. As she talked about Stan and her relationship with him, and as she unfolded how she had been coping over the weeks and months of loss she had already experienced, it seemed to me that she was managing pretty well. The stages of grief were typical. The loss had been devastating but the stream of life had begun to flow again. The direction of the flow was indeed different, and she was dealing with that. There was little I could tell her that was new. Images such as the stream and the boulder did not need to be used. That would have been for an earlier stage. She was past that. She seemed to be doing well.

In the midst of her sharing with me, she stopped and sat silent for a long time. Then she began to cry. Not sobbing, not hysteria, not brokenness, but sorrow from deep within her. Down the dignified, composed face, rolled big, glistening tears. There was beauty in what I was watching. But there was also deep, heartfelt grief. And slowly, with the tears still falling, she spoke: 'I miss him so much. He was everything to me, my husband, a father to our children, my lover, my constant companion, my best friend. I have lost everything that makes my life have meaning. I can think of nothing else. I get by with other people. I keep up for my daughters and their families. I socialise. I go to church. I cope. But when I am alone, I cry and cry. Oh how I miss him, how I miss him.'

I cried with Rita, such was the passion of her loss. I knelt beside her and held her hands. We cried together, and waited, in silence, till the tears subsided. I do not know how long this episode lasted. But I do know how deep it was.

When the tears were over, and I had returned to my seat, Rita looked me straight in the eye, and asked, 'Will I ever get over Stan's death?' 'No,' I replied, 'you won't.' 'Will it ever make sense, then? Will I ever be able to live with it?' 'Yes,' I replied, 'you will.' And we talked about perspective, and moving on, and the like. And all the while I was searching my mind for another picture, an image which would help us understand together what was happening.

My gaze fell on my painting on the wall. My eye was drawn to the damaged part. And I shared this exploration with Rita, and word for word, as far as I can recall it, I share it with you.

Rising from my chair, I went over to the picture. I told Rita about where the painting had come from, and how it had got damaged. And I pointed out the mark to her. I went right up close to the picture, right up against the mark. 'Rita,' I said, 'what is happening is that you are this close to the damage Stanley's death has caused in the picture of your life. You are this close. All you can see is the damage. You are transfixed by it. You are angry at it, distressed by it. It is the focus of your whole being. The idyllic picture of your life has been damaged, through no fault of your own. There is a mark where there should be no mark. And you cannot take your eyes off the flaw.' I paused to let the silence run. 'But,' I continued after a while, 'in time, slowly and steadily, you will stand back from the painting.'

And as I spoke, I moved slowly backwards. 'As you move, you will still keep your eyes on the damage. It will still take your attention, you will remain transfixed by it, because it will not go away. It has changed the picture for ever. But as you move back, you see more of the picture. It is inevitable. The rest of it will come into focus again. Familiar sections, parts of beauty and colour and life, areas of love and wonder, things you have not seen for a while because you have been so close to the damaged section, will come into view again. So you will look at them, see them in their place, get the whole thing in perspective.' Once again I paused. 'And the flaw will remain, to take your attention again from time to time, to be moved close to, to be studied once more in detail, and even to make you angry and distressed again. But now it is clearly surrounded by the rest of life, which can still have meaning and beauty and form.'

I looked at Rita, and she had begun to cry again. But now she smiled through her tears. And she nodded. She said nothing. She just nodded and smiled. She had understood.

I met Rita again a little while ago. We greeted each other warmly. We spent a while catching up with each other. And, before we parted, she said, 'Do you remember what you shared with me about your damaged painting?' I nodded. 'Well,' she continued, 'you were right. It is about perspective. I still look at the damage to my picture, and I get angry, and I get sad. But there is a lot in the rest of the picture that makes me remember other things, that makes me feel warm inside, that makes me smile again and again.'

The important issue here for me is facing the reality that the mark on the painting cannot be erased. Just as the boulder remains lodged in its place in the stream, never to be removed, such that the flow has to take a different course, so the damaged mark remains on the painting for the rest of the painting to contain it for ever and absorb it into its form and colour and life.

I spoke with a widow recently who reminded me that it was four years since her husband had died. She told me that on the previous Sunday she had broken down in church and couldn't hold back the tears. She was angry with herself. She had been doing fine. She hadn't fallen out with the children. She had no problems at work. It wasn't PMT. She was even enjoying the service – till they got to the blessing sung at the end of a baptism. It is an emotional enough moment at the best of times, but on this occasion she dissolved into uncontrollable tears. She was back at the death of her husband, back feeling alone with the children, back with the brokenness and the pain and the anger.

She said that she was so overcome that she had to leave, embarrassed by her tears, not wanting to cause any distress to those around her, not wishing to disrupt the baptism. She knew that this would happen from time to time. She had read the books on the grief process, she had been to our meetings, she had even helped others through their bereavements. But four years on? Part of her was panicking, saying, 'It's time this shouldn't be happening,' that it was unacceptable, that something was wrong.

Since the death of my father – and more recently the loss of my wife's father, the final grandparent of our children – I know what this is like, because I have been in the same situation. I know how it felt for her. For me it fell apart during a drama on television where I could identify closely with a relative facing the death of a loved one. What was happening to that widow was that her attention had been drawn, when she least expected it, to the damage, the flaw, the pain of the death of her life-partner. It was the offence of the spoiled painting that had caused her to hurt once more.

The trouble is that memories of the past are so much part of you that they pop up from time to time, often when they are least expected – a fragment of music; a silly, personal recollection; a smell; a letter addressed to the person who has died; an old photo; a line of a hymn – and bang, emotion overwhelms you again. You can't eradicate times like that any more than you can rub out the memory of the person who has gone. So every so often something happens to remind you of the damage to the painting, and you hurt until your perspective is regained and you see the damage once again absorbed by the whole picture.

That is what happened with Rita. Her horizons had altered again – slowly, often too slowly for her wishes – over time. Now she could see the bigger picture once more. And what was still there were the things that would last: the identity, the completeness, of the man she loved.

My damaged painting is still hanging in my office as I write this chapter. Sometimes when I'm at my desk I glance over my shoulder to look at it. And often now the way the light falls on the picture means that I can't make out the flaw at all. I know it is there, but I would have to look hard to find it. So I just sit for a moment and enjoy the beauty the evening light creates on the rest of a beautiful painting.

I end this chapter with a final thought. The picture shared with me by a bereaved person, with its flaws and its beauty, is unique to that individual. Of course there are familiar aspects to the grief process, predictable periods that one can watch for and guide people through, well documented stages which have to be worked with and understood. But the patterns of grief, the time it takes for each stage to be dealt with, and indeed the methodology utilised by people to work through the process of bereavement have to remain unique. The picture is their own.

I recall being upset with a doctor who clearly felt that the fact that a widow still had her husband's toothbrush in its holder above the wash-hand basin was an indication of abnormal grief. She had been widowed for 18 months. In his view the toothbrush was a sign that she was unable to let her husband go, that she was stuck, in denial, grieving abnormally, or whatever. If he had bothered to listen to her, to be drawn into her picture, he would have learned a different story. She wasn't stuck at all. The toothbrush was simply part of the familiar layout of the bathroom, a piece of her picture. Keeping it in place was one of the ways she coped.

It is easy to judge, to feel, 'Well, if that was me, I wouldn't be doing things that way.' But we are not, and cannot be, the person who is bereaved. Their picture is their picture. It is our task to learn from it and to seek to understand – 'take a walk under my skies' as James Keelaghan has written.

When one of my children was four years old and in nursery school, I went one day to collect her and take her home. She had been painting, as children do, and had 'done a picture for Daddy'. When she saw me arrive, she bounded up to me with great enthusiasm, 'Daddy, Daddy, I've painted you a picture.' I took the painting from her. It was still wet and, as a typical child's painting, had colours everywhere, with no shape I could discern, representing nothing I could understand. 'What's this?' I asked. Just then a buxom nursery assistant whom I knew well came along. She put a big arm round my shoulder. 'A word, Mr Gordon ...,' she suggested. And taking me aside she offered me, in a few moments, a lesson I have never forgotten. 'Never,' she said, 'ask a child "What's that?" when they have done something for you. Because that's a judgement. It tells the child that you don't understand, that you are being critical, or even that they have failed to communicate the message of their painting to you. Instead say, "Tell me about your painting" or "What's happening in your picture?" and you will get the story and the meaning of what they have done. You will be inviting them to take you into their world. You will be communicating that you are prepared to listen and to understand the picture they have painted.'

I have remembered that lesson as I have worked with many people who are bereaved, in the childlike, vulnerable state bereavement brings. So I have said often, 'Tell me what's happening in your picture,' and have had the privilege of being drawn into some wonderful paintings, each one different from the others, but each with a story to tell, a uniqueness to be understood, and a beauty to be valued.

How long?

How long has this to be?
How long am I to be consumed by this –
this pain,
this loss,
this separation?
How long am I to be drawn,
day after day,
minute by painful minute,
to its dreadful happening?
How long to weep,
and know that weeping as a constant companion?
How long, my God, how long?

How often has this to be?
How often am I to be reminded
of this parting,
when I do not want to be,
I do not expect to be?
How often will a look
a smell
a sound

drag me back to look
and to know again the pain?
How often, my God, how often?

How unfair has this to be?
How unfair to lose him now,
when so much was promised,
planned,
expected,
when so much was done to share and love,
believing it could last and last?
How unfair
to see no more the light and shade of living
but only that one dark place
where all was lost
in your departing?
How unfair, my God, how unfair?

Fourteen

The untidy drawer

Canst thou not minister to a mind diseas'd,
Pluck from the memory a rooted sorrow,
Raze out the written troubles of the brain,
And with some sweet oblivious antidote
Cleanse the stuff'd bosom of that perilous stuff
Which weighs upon the heart?
Shakespeare: Macbeth

Everything must be done in a proper and orderly way.
1 Corinthians 14:40

Visits to my grandmother, which were a familiar part of our family life when I was a child, were for a small boy filled with wonder and delight. My granny and grandpa seemed to me – and were, in fact – from a different age. From the west coast of Scotland, having worked on farms all their days, and rooted in Glasgow culture and attitudes, they were always fascinating people. Their accent was quite different from the Highland lilt I was familiar with. Different words were used, deriving as they did from a mixture of broad Scots and the Glasgow vernacular. Ways of doing things, the food we ate, even the smell of the house were all different, full of wonder and newness for an inquisitive and interested child.

I recall the fascination of watching my granny making a 'clootie dumpling', delighting in placing the silver coins in the bowl knowing I would find them later in the finished article (as if they were buried treasure I never suspected would be there). I remember the kitchen being filled with a wonderful smell, and the dumpling being carried in triumph from the kitchen to steam before a blazing fire to create its outer skin, shiny and inviting.

Even yet I can picture my grandpa, ensconced in his favourite chair by the fire, bottle of beer on one side, ash-tray and pipe on the other. I can see him shaking with his Parkinson's disease ('His nerves got shot when he was tossed by a bull,' my granny would relate with relish), shaking ever more wildly when he was excited by a boxing match on that fascinating 14-inch, black-and-white TV set in the corner. I can hear the ever-rising sound of the box of Swan Vesta matches held tightly in the hand, now in the excitement being shaken as frenetically as maracas in a samba band, till, when they reached their crescendo, my granny would shout, 'Would you put the bloody matches down, man. I cannae hear masel' think!'

I will never forget the rituals of the New Year gatherings. There were the dumpling and the black bun (Why only at New Year were such wonderful treats brought out?), the songs when the drink had flowed (the same songs every year sung in the same order by the same people), the ginger wine (for the children!) which seared a track down the back of a small boy's throat even though he felt so grown up drinking like the adults did.

But most of all, amidst all that was fascinating in this wonderful world of 'going to my granny's', I remember the drawer in the kitchen table. This drawer, above all else, was what going-to-granny's was all about. This was a drawer the very opening of which led to a land of magic, of fascination, of excitement. It was a drawer the likes of which I had never seen, and which no adult appeared concerned that a child should enter.

Into this drawer, over many years, things had been thrown, maybe not Shakespeare's 'perilous stuff', but stuff none the less – fascinating stuff, different stuff, wonderful stuff – and all, it appeared to me, solely for my amusement and delight!

This was the drawer with the broken watch, the metal ruler, the flat joiner's pencil. (Why weren't pencils at school as fun as this?)

This was the drawer with the green ration-book, the foreign stamps with the wonderful pictures, the rubber washers from the screw-tops from lemonade bottles. This was the drawer with the marbles, the brass lighter with no fuel, the tattered cigarette cards with faded, dog-eared images of famous football players and cricketing legends. This was the drawer with the brass curtain rings, the broken coat-hook, the packet of carpet-tacks. This was the drawer with the set of false teeth, the whistle with no pea, the empty tobacco tin with its wonderful smell.

This was the drawer in my granny's kitchen table, a veritable treasure trove, giving hours of happy entertainment to a little boy. This was the place of fun, of imagination, of discovery. This, above all else, was what made going-to-granny's worthwhile.

But not so for my granny! For while she was more than content, with the rest of the family, to see me happily amused and therefore out from under their feet when they did their grown-up things, she would get more than mildly irritated when things would be taken out of the drawer and left lying about when I was bored with them. Finding a pair of false teeth on the kitchen table or standing on a stray marble in the hall, she would be heard shouting: 'Tom, where on earth did you get this?' She knew full well, of course, and would retrieve the offending item and return it to its Aladdin's cave, with the rest of the collection of oddments and treasures.

And that's just the point. For her, and for the other grown-ups, this drawer was no treasure trove, no gateway to imaginative wonders and joys. It was simply a place to tidy things away when there was nowhere else to put them – things that had no place of their own, to be looked at later, to be sorted, matched, reused, or whatever, when the time came. But not just now. So to keep the place tidy – or at least tidy enough for others to feel the house was in order – she had her drawer, and anything and everything was jammed in there. This was the place where my granny put her stuff!

No adult was permitted access. Indeed, no adult would have wanted access to such a jumbled mess. The inquisitive child asked no questions and made no judgements regarding the state and contents of the drawer, content simply to play and enjoy. For adults, however, it was my granny's private place, where things got put away, to be returned to – or, more often, not – when the drawer was full to overflowing.

Through the years I have come to realise that my granny was not unique! My mother also had such a drawer. For her it was in the sideboard in the living room. It was the place, I recall, where the mouth-organ was kept. But that was all I was allowed to retrieve from that drawer, as my mother made it quite clear that the rest was not to be touched. What was in there that could be so important, so private? What secrets did this drawer contain? I never knew, because the drawer – itself full to overflowing – was always my mother's drawer, filled with my mother's stuff, her own private space.

Now I have a drawer like that. Indeed, I have to confess, I have several. One is in my bedside table – oh, I shudder to think what is in there: it's such a long time since I had a good look ... Another is in a cupboard in the garage – different stuff, same kind of drawer. Indeed, human nature being what it is – and I don't think my granny or my mother or myself are that different from the rest of humanity! – I know we must all have such a drawer, that place where things get put, jammed, stuffed, to get them out of the way, to tidy the place, to keep them safe till we have time to look at them, to sort them, to order them, to fix them, to discard them – but always later on. We never get around to it, though, or at least not often. And day after day, week after week, more and more things get stuffed in, till sometimes the drawer is full to overflowing, and might even be hard to open. What are we to do then?

The task, if we are sensible and can put our mind to it, is to begin a sorting process: to clear the kitchen table, cover it with newspaper, tip out the drawer to see what's there, and start to sort it out. But which of us does that? It is too time-consuming, and there always seem to be better, more pressing things to do. It is too complicated, requiring thoroughness, thoughtfulness, decisions. It requires us to be somewhat self-critical. (Why did I ever let this drawer get into such a mess in the first place?) So the task of tidying the drawer is something we never quite get around to. And the drawer is left as always, stuffed to overflowing.

Until, that is, the crisis comes, and we have no choice. Crisis? Well, what if the drawer is so full you have nowhere to put anything else until you clear some space? What if you have to find something – the letter, the matching earring, the address you scribbled down on a scrap of paper – and you need it now and it's probably in that drawer? What if … Then you have no choice, and the tense, difficult task of doing what you have put off doing for so long has to begin. The contents of the drawer have to be sorted – at last.

The image of the kitchen-table drawer is one which I keep in the forefront of my mind in the work I do with patients and family members, and indeed sometimes with staff too, as they seek my time in looking at the issues that matter to them. I would be considered to be an experienced minister. I am well versed in the role of a hospice chaplain. I have trained in listening skills, counselling techniques, psychological insights. But I am not, and will not be in this setting, a counsellor. Counselling, entering into a long-term, therapeutic relationship with a client, has its place in providing a professional framework in which people can work through their crises and problems. Indeed, when the need arises, it is often appropriate to refer people from this setting – particularly in the journey of bereavement – to a counselling agency so that long-term work can be embarked upon. But my role as hospice chaplain is not to be a guru, a therapist or a counsellor for people with complicated and long-standing needs. My role is to help them sort what's in their kitchen drawer!

Lorna was a young, attractive woman whose husband, Donald, had died in our hospice after a short and trying illness. She and Donald had three children, Faith aged 4, John aged 7 and Sophie aged 9. The shortness of Donald's illness, the emaciated condition of his body before death, and the planning and coping with the funeral had left the family drained and confused. Issues of coping with the children, Lorna's own health (she had lost a lot of weight in a very short time during Donald's illness), the deep sorrow of both Lorna and Donald's parents were all hard to bear. The journey of grief and loss was a painful one indeed.

Lorna came to our bereavement support meetings for several months – and she did very well. Slowly, with insight and commitment, listening and talking, finding resources within herself she did not believe she had, she worked at the issues. She would take advice, guidance and reassurance, go away and apply them, and come back and reflect on her journey of bereavement once more. Eventually, she went back to work. She regained the weight she had lost. She found some of her old vivacity. As far as we could see things were progressing fine.

One evening, at the conclusion of our support meeting, Lorna took me aside. 'Can I come to see you by myself?' she asked. I was puzzled. I had never thought there was anything we had been missing in dealing with Lorna. What could she want time for on her own? However, subduing my natural curiosity, I arranged to meet her later in the week. And in my office Lorna began to talk about the journey of loss and how she was coping. Some parts I had heard before and some bits were new – but there was more. There was much more. There were references to her relationships with her parents, issues from childhood, self-esteem and the like. There was an issue around the loss of her husband as her sexual partner – something she could never have shared with a group of people. There were questions about God, never raised before but which she was feeling would not go away, and she had no one to air them with and have them taken seriously. There were lots of other bits and pieces, in no particular order, that came tumbling out too. In short, there was a lot of 'stuff', accumulated over a long time, put away with other stuff because there wasn't the necessity or the energy or the commitment or the confidence to look at it at the time. But now? Now there was too much stuff. The big issues of dealing with death made the drawer too full, even though it had been full enough to start with! Now it was all tumbling out. It was demanding to be sorted through.

Lorna had discovered that the drawer in her kitchen table needed to be looked at. She had no choice, she confessed. It was now or never – and if it was never, could she live with this mess all her life without it 'doing her head in', as she put it? And so we made a deal – and I said this to her just as I am setting it out here – that I would not be her therapist because, from my assessment of her circumstances, that was not what she needed. (And if she did, we would decide that later and look at it when it was necessary.) She didn't, to my view, have a 'problem'. But I said I would be prepared to be the person who could help with the sorting of the stuff in her kitchen-table drawer. I would spend time with her, clearing the table, spreading out the newspaper and sorting through the contents.

And that's just what we did. We set ourselves three weeks to do it, and we agreed to assess things at the end of three weeks to see if we needed more time. So we had three hour-and-a-half sessions, and carefully we sorted the contents of the drawer. We looked at different things. Some were hard to pick up and think about and some were funny. Some could be dealt with quickly, and some took a long time. Some were thrown away, considered now to be over-and-done-with; some – cherished, important things – were carefully examined and put back. Some were grouped together, some were fixed and renewed. And slowly, one by one, the things in the drawer were sorted through. In the end, we didn't need any longer than the three weeks. The drawer was tidy to Lorna's satisfaction. She now knew what was there. The drawer could be opened again when she needed to open it, and she would not require any assistance to do so. The fear of the unknown had gone. Confidence had returned. The sorting had worked.

For me, setting out a 'contract' in a relationship such as this and using the image of the drawer did a number of things. Firstly, it reminded Lorna and myself that the drawer and its contents were, and always would be, hers and not mine. I could help her with the sorting. I could be with her in the scary moments and I could share the enjoyment of the funny things. But I would not take on the responsibility of doing the sorting. That was for her to do. She would have to go on living with the drawer.

Secondly, it gave a time limit and a framework for our work together. There was no commitment to a long-term relationship. It was, I suppose, akin to what has become known as 'brief counselling', because that was all that was required.

Thirdly, it gave Lorna a picture with which she could go on working on her own. Of course there would be things she would go on stuffing into her drawer. That's part of the journey of life. (My granny taught me that at an early age!) But now she had the confidence to return to the drawer on occasions before the next crisis arose – before the drawer was too full to open, or something had got lost, or the contents were tumbling out – and work at the process some more, before closing the drawer for another while.

And finally – just like working in William's attic – it reminded me that I have a drawer too, full of my stuff. And it's high time I got the table cleared and started working on that!

As I write this and reflect on the image of the drawer and my sessions with Lorna – and many others over the years – I am intrigued that I have said little about the actual issues Lorna raised with me, the specific contents of her untidy drawer. It is not that they didn't matter at the time or that I didn't take them seriously. It is just that they don't matter now. They have been put away for Lorna to live with and deal with, until such time as she may need me or some-one else to help with another sorting process.

Each drawer is unique, to be owned, dealt with, added to, sorted as appropriate to the individual concerned. And the wonderful thing is this: hidden deep in every drawer, like the treasures in a drawer in a granny's kitchen table, there are some wonderful things, magic things, exciting things, things long since forgotten, buried deep under a pile of other 'stuff' that 'weighs upon the heart', that might never be found again or brought out with renewed pleasure unless the sorting begins.

What follows is a letter sent to me some years ago. In it you will see how one person made use of the image in this chapter. But she is not unique. We all have an untidy drawer – or maybe more than one! What is it in your drawer that you need to think about tidying? Do you need to do it now? Who do you need to help you? And what letter would you write when the tidying had begun?

Dear Tom

It's nearly a year now since Dad died, and I'm only just getting round to clearing out his stuff. I couldn't face it at the beginning. It was all too final, too dismissive of a long and full life. My brother kept nagging me to get on with it. But you know Bob, he always wants to get things over and done with ASAP. But I couldn't face it. It was too much.

And, anyway, I remembered what you said about my own dressing-table drawer. I don't know if you remember our conversation – I'm sure you speak to so many people – but I remember it very well. And so I decided to use the time to do my own sorting before I started on my Dad's. So I bought a big exercise book and I started to write things down – stuff from childhood, things that began as vague memories and all of a sudden became vivid again. I went back to the village where I was born and walked down familiar streets. I wrote to a school friend I hadn't seen in years and suggested we get back in touch again – and she wrote back and we're meeting up next weekend! *Yes!* I began to let go of some worries I'd been putting off dealing with for ages; I confided in a close friend, and she was really helpful – you know, just listening and letting me prattle – and you know I'm good at that! I cried a lot – an awful lot – my exercise book has more tear stains on it than anyone will ever know. I gave Eric a huge hug when he came home from work the other day and I told him I loved him – and he didn't know what had hit him! He's lovely and I love him to bits. He's been so patient with me, though I'm sure he doesn't really understand what I've been working on.

So, I sorted my drawer, and it was hard. I thought of phoning you often, but I didn't. Maybe I should have done. Maybe the sorting would have been easier, quicker. I don't know. But I just struggled on. And, you know, it's helped a lot – an awful lot. Why didn't I do it before? But we don't do we? It's not that I've got it all done. Goodness, there's *years* of stuff to sort out! But I've done enough for now. At least I can get the drawer shut again!

So, now, I've been able to get on with my Dad's stuff too – a different kind of sorting, but still to be done with time and care. I'm getting there with that as well. So, thank you – for reading this ramble for one thing. But for telling me about your granny's table drawer when I was struggling with Dad's death. It really helped. I'll be in touch soon. But I wanted to let you know how I was getting on. You can put this letter in your table drawer – provided it's tidy enough to have some space left! Sorry – that's very cheeky.

I wish you well with all your work. Please tell the nurses I'm asking for them. And thank you all once more for looking after Dad.

Much love
Jane

Fifteen

Climbing the rock face

Fain would I climb, yet fear I to fall
Sir Walter Raleigh: Line written on a window pane

To cry, 'Hold! Hold'
Shakespeare: Macbeth

Someone once said – and I think it might even have been me in a time of great angst! – that being a parent is one of the few things in life for which you have no training. Yes, there are models of good parenting to follow, there are books to read and there are discussions to be entered into. But for most of us, most of the time, it is a matter of intuition, doing the best we can with the circumstances we are facing, and hoping we will get it right. Thankfully, it turns out OK – well, most of the time, anyway. But the processes are not without their anxieties, tensions and worries and, as any parent will know, bringing up children has its times of trauma and disaster.

As I indicated earlier, Mary and I have three children who, at the time of writing this, are all in their twenties. They are close together in age – our third was born six months before the eldest's fourth birthday – and when they were little we struggled with a succession of 'Terrible Twos' and the like. When they were in their teens and we worked and socialised with others who had younger children, we were often asked – as people sought to draw upon the wisdom of our maturer years! – 'Does it get any better?' to which I would always reply: 'No, not better, just different!'

In my understanding of parenting, that is just the point – there has to be an adjustment to the different stages a child goes through, and ideally it is an adjustment from both sides, so that family life can deal with the new experiences and traumas that growing up brings. Such is the pain and the joy of being a father or a mother. Such is the hard work that never seems to diminish.

And such was the thought process that once again came to mind when I sat down with my second daughter a year or so ago. She had not long finished college, having achieved a qualification in child care and education, but she wasn't at all sure about what she wanted to do next. Tying herself down to a 'career' didn't seem right at this stage as there were so many ideas buzzing around in her head – voluntary work, working abroad, doing more study, travelling, and a hundred-and-one other things – and she couldn't figure which way to go. She had taken a job as a barmaid while she was 'reviewing her future', so that she had some money to live on. And she was living at home.

Now, therein is an example of my retort, 'No, it doesn't get better, it just gets different!' For this living-at-home was different, a new phase which required adjustment all round and patience and toler-ance in large measures. Can Radio 1 find a peaceful coexistence with Radio 2 – when both are played at the same time and, of course, with one much louder than the other? Can regular meal times accommodate flexible eating – 'No, I don't know when I'll be in. Keep something for me if you like.' Can reasonably early-bedders cope with late night TV and early-morning banging of doors?

You get the picture? Most of the time it was fine. Sometimes it wasn't too good. And occasionally it was downright intolerable – and not just for us, for we are far from being saintly parents, but for our daughter, and her younger brother who was also staying at home, as she struggled to understand what to her must have been strange habits and patterns of living.

Through it all, we talked. Thank God, we talked! Sometimes it was in snatched conversations, occasionally communication was through the white message-board outside the kitchen, often the talk would be into the wee, small hours of the morning. But we talked. And in that very fact was salvation for all of us, and the continuation of a framework for dealing with the ups and downs of family life.

One evening, when we were all in together for once and watching the same TV programme, my daughter leaned over to me and said: 'Dad, we need to talk!' 'Now?' I asked. 'Yes please,' she replied. So, while the others strained to keep up with the TV programme, we talked. And we talked about the future.

She wanted to move out – something we had talked about on and off for a number of months – and share a flat with friends. There were possibilities on the horizon and they were being clarified even as we spoke. She was also unhappy in her job. She was feeling unfulfilled and unaffirmed in the pub, and was thinking about moving to another pub where she felt she would be happier. She was looking through the job pages of the local paper and writing off to various places to explore longer-term employment or voluntary commitments. She was talking about taking time out from everything to go to work on Iona with the Community there. She was excited about some things, unclear about different parts, and terrified of others.

So we talked. And as we did so I saw a young woman trying to move on, to take another step in her own growth and development. I saw a young woman not sure which step to take first. I saw a young woman fearful of coming crashing down if there was too much happening at once. And I saw in my mind a climber on a rock face.

Now, my daughter has no aspirations to be a climber. Indeed, nor have I. But I have watched with fascination and much admiration climbers going about their business – from the Old Man of Hoy to the north face of the Eiger, from practice climbs in an indoor climbing school to expeditions to Everest and the like. And I recall this advice from a climbing programme on TV many years ago: When you climb, in order to stay safe, you should have three points of contact with the rock face at any one time. Move a hand to find a new handhold, and keep two feet and one hand where they are, firm and secure. Move a foot up on to a new ledge, but keep holding on with two hands and the other foot remaining solid where it is. Three points of contact all the time. Only move one upwards or downwards or outwards at any one time. Take two points of contact off the rock face, and you are foolhardy and in grave danger. Take three points off and … well …

So I shared this with my daughter. Trying to do too much at once was where the fear of falling came from, I suggested. Why not think about changing one thing at a time. Move into your flat, but keep the job in the pub for now and see how it goes. Then, when you are settled in the flat – and that point of contact is once again secure to the rock face – then you can look at changing jobs and move another point of contact to a new, secure hold. Get the flat and the job secure, and that gives you a firm starting point for the next move – a permanent job, moving away, or wherever the explorations take you – another new handhold or foothold which takes you a little bit further on the climb.

She nodded sagely. (Sometimes what a father says makes sense!) And this image seemed to do just that – it made sense. It created for her a picture into which she could place herself. It gave her a concept with which we would be able to break down the many decisions which were causing the anxiety and work on one of them at a time.

We do not have the luxury all the time of being able to be as clear as this. Often many decisions have to be made at the same time – it is not uncommon for a marriage, a change of job and a house move all to be dealt with at once. Three major changes? Three points of contact being moved off the rock face to find new holds? No wonder people get stressed!

However, when we do have to face change and make decisions about moving on following, for example, a major life event, then the picture of the climber on the rock face can be a helpful one.

So my daughter moved into a flat. And, at the time of writing this, she is using that new, secure place in her life as a foundation from which to explore other things – one move at a time.

To be honest, I don't know where the picture came from or why it was in my mind at that time. It just seemed to pop up out of nowhere. (What's that bit in the Bible about God giving us the right things to say at the right time?) Anyway, from wherever it came, it seemed to work.

And having utilised this picture with my daughter in her circumstances, I mulled it over and begun tentatively to offer it to people in my work setting.

I talked recently with Mandy, a young widow with whom I had worked on bereavement issues for some time. She had done well, carefully working through the different stages and taking advice and guidance from myself and others. In time, I had done as much with her as I was able, and we went our separate ways. I often wondered how she was getting on, and then one day I met her at a social function. There she was, looking great, and with a new man on her arm. She told me how things had been going. She had retrained in computers and had settled in a good job. Three years after her husband died she sold their flat and bought a new house out of town. And now she had a 'new fella' and life was good. When her 'fella' had slipped off to the bar, Mandy told me that in the beginning – well, after a reasonable time as a widow – she became aware of friends trying to 'fix her up' with a succession of 'fellas' which she just wasn't ready for. 'Not that some of them weren't very fanciable,' she smiled … It's just that she wasn't ready to have a new relationship at that point. But now that job and house were sorted out, now that she was sure her moves had given her stability again, she was ready to give her 'fella' her best shot. And I told her that he was a very lucky guy!

Mandy had been working with the image of the climber on the rock face and she didn't even know she was doing it.

Some years ago, after I had led a seminar at a local church on issues of grief and loss, I had a conversation with Tim, one of the church's pastoral care group. He told me as we talked together about his bereavement journey that he had stopped going to church. Not that he didn't want to and, indeed, not that he didn't need to. But it was just too hard. He couldn't get over the emotion, and he felt he was letting himself, his pastor, his congregation and his God down. He would watch 'Songs of Praise' and TV church services, and weep buckets. But at least no one saw him like that. It was private. So going to church was out for now.

What he had done, however, was to buy a season ticket for his local football team – something he hadn't been able to do for years because he had been his wife's main carer during her illness. Why was he able to do this, he asked, when he couldn't go to church? What kind of Christian was he when he could handle a secular pursuit and put energy into that and not be able to be committed to worship on a Sunday?

We talked round this and many other issues, and I suggested to him that he shouldn't worry about it. I put him on his rock face. I reckoned that getting back behind his team, meeting with pals, having a day out for himself, was enough for now. And, anyway, his football team needed all the support they could get!

Was I right? Should I have pushed him into working through the struggle with going to church? Well, maybe I should. But I reckoned that he needed to get firm on the rock face before he stressed himself with something else. One thing at a time ...

I was conducting a funeral service recently and I saw Tim in the congregation – three years or so after we had spoken together. He came to speak with me afterwards, and he told me he was doing well. I tentatively asked him about church. He smiled and told me he was going regularly again, and had been for the past year. It felt good to have got that sorted out once more. But it had had to take time – although, he confessed, it hadn't changed the fortunes of his football team one iota!

So climbing the rock face is a slow and careful process. Don't take too many risks when you don't have to. Take time – and care – to get it right, and as Tim and Mandy and my lovely daughter will tell you, your progress will still go on.

I'm stuck

It is so slow, this journey of change –
so much to think about
so much to do
so much to decide
so much …

I'm stuck.
Will it always be like this –
the uncertainty,
the fear,
the loneliness?

I don't know where to begin,
what to change,
what to tackle first,
what to try.

I'm so alone.
Has anyone felt like this before?
Surely no one will know
or understand
or appreciate
what this is like for me?

It seems so insurmountable
this climb
out of my pit of despair,
so impossible,
so incredible.
What's the point of even trying?

I can't hold on any more.
I'm letting go.
I'll fall,
I'll fail.
I'll never live again.

*

But there,
there,
above me –
what's that?
A hold?
A jutting rock
that might …
just
possibly …
be within my reach?
Yes …
yes …
I … can … just … make … it …

My God,
but that was hard,
the attempt,
the effort,
the desire to try.

But now,
this rock has a different feel,
different shape,

different grip,
different view …
Why do I feel different too?

So, what next?
There …
there …
a little ledge?
Another try,
another move,
another inch …

My God,
would you believe it?
I'm really climbing,
me,
upwards …
now …

One thing at a time!

Here's an exercise we so often do in our heads, or in our prayers, or in discussion with trusted people. Try committing it to paper and create a picture of this process for yourself.

- Find yourself a quiet place, away from distractions.

- Sit down in a comfortable place with a notebook or a blank sheet of paper.

- Spend some time thinking about the things in your present life that are dependable, firm and steady, which you feel support you in what you are doing. Perhaps it's a relationship, a job, the place you stay, your family, a church, a qualification, your faith.

- Write them down.

- Ponder each one, think about its purpose, how long it has been good for you, the people who provide it, the places where it happens.

- Pray about each one, with gratitude, with pleasure, with purpose.

- Now spend some time thinking about the things that are changing in your life, the parts that are unsteady, from which you have to firm up again or from which you need to move on. Maybe it will be a change of job, moving house, starting or ending a relationship, saying sorry to someone you love, taking up a college course, sorting out your faith.

- Write them down.

- Think through each one, why it is important, what needs to be changed, how you are feeling, apprehensions about the future.

- Pray about each one, remembering that apprehensions and fears are as much part of living as certainties and gratitude.

- Now draw yourself a rock face – just a simple square on the paper will do – and on the bottom half write in the things you are sure of, the firm footholds of your life. Think about the top three of these, the ones that are most important, most firm, and put these together, like three hand and footholds on the rock.

- Now, from your list of changes, take the two or three that are most important, the ones that are pressing to be dealt with first, which are causing you most anxiety. Write them on the rock face too, the most worrying ones quite close to the most firm ones.

- Now draw a line between the firm footholds and handholds and the one change you feel you have to tackle first. Along that line, write what you have to do to make that change happen, and when you are going to reach for it.

- Have a go at using your firm hold to reach for the new one.

- Keep your lists and your picture of the rock face. Go back and do the exercise again when your new position is secure. Work out your next move. And see how you are progressing upwards, one hold at a time!

Sixteen

The table

A child should always say what's true,
And speak when he is spoken to,
And behave mannerly at table:
At least as far as he is able.
Robert Louis Stevenson: A Child's Garden of Verse

Good people all, of every sort,
Give ear unto my song;
And if you find it wond'rous short,
It cannot hold you long
Oliver Goldsmith: Elegy on the Death of a Mad Dog

John Simpson, writing of his experiences as a BBC foreign corre-spondent, tells of how finding an outlet for his journalistic skills, as well as his TV reporting, was immensely therapeutic for him. In addition to the feeling of independence and freedom his writing gave him, he says this of the value of his work for *The Spectator* and *The Sunday Telegraph*:

Writing did something else for me. I found it cauterised whatever emotional wounds I suffered in my travels … Once these experiences were honestly set down on paper and the article was faxed to London, that was effectively the end of it. I would continue to feel sorrow or pity, but the memories no longer seemed to inflame the layers of my subconscious mind like a kind of mental cellulitis.

In part, I know what John Simpson means. I have always been a storyteller, and the recounting of crazy tales and incidents with fasci-nating people has always been a therapy for me. For one thing, it has allowed me to reflect, to examine, and to let go of some of the madness and pain.

But, in one particular way I would differ from Simpson's analysis. The telling of stories, and the bringing back to mind of the people involved (and now writing down some reflections on them) is not for me about letting them go, and it is certainly not the end of it. For in a very real sense I am still 'inflamed' by the people about whom I write and about whom I speak. Bringing them to mind in written word or spoken voice serves to allow me to be near them once more, and to learn again from their involvement with me.

So the people of whom I have written, and the many more whose stories are not yet committed to paper, are, if you like, part of what I now am. They are not simply characters of stories inhabiting the pages of a book. They are fundamentally part of me.

What I have given them, I hope, has been of value. What they have given me, of insight, compassion, tolerance, strength, faith, acceptance and depth, is of much greater value. Their rich resources remain with me to allow me to make something more available to others.

As a Church of Scotland minister, I had to undergo, through our Presbyterian system, what are known as 'Trials for Licence' when I was preparing for my ministry. This meant an examination by Presbytery in matters of Church Law and Doctrine, as well as preaching before representatives of the Presbytery and being 'critted' afterwards on my conduct of worship and the content of the sermon. 'Trial' was certainly a good description, as it was an ordeal all round!

Most of my Trials for Licence went past in a blur and it is now no more than a hazy memory. But two things remain with me from thirty years ago – the first is a criticism from a minister from Presbytery that I had not prayed for the Queen and her Royal Household. And the second – communicated to me with even more passion than the first – was that I had omitted to give thanks for the 'blessed departed' or the Communion of Saints.

I suppose as a young trainee minister I thought I knew better than an old hand. I understood, I think, the issue about the royal family. But the criticism of the omission of a reference to the Communion of Saints somehow passed me by, confined to the bin marked 'good advice from wiser people' that I did not recognise for its worth and value at the time.

As years of ministry have passed, I have come to realise that that old minister was quite correct. And so the concept of the Communion of Saints, the 'blessed departed', has become increasingly important over the years. This is not because it is an idea to which I feel I have to subscribe to make me a 'proper' minister, but because it matters in my soul to carry with me the countless numbers of people who have touched me deeply through the years with their love, their insights and the value of their lives.

Nowhere is that more true than in my present work as a hospice chaplain. I have said already that I have gained more from the people I have met along the way than I have ever given. I am the richer for their interactions with me, and I am the better for the memories I have of them.

In another of his thoughtful songs, Tom Paxton talks about faces and places which leave 'indelible traces' on the soul of a person. Indelible traces on my soul – from Bobby and Andy, from Rita and Cathie, from Violet and William, and countless others who are no longer names, but vague impressions, hazy memories, snatched recollections – and the traces they have left will never be erased.

So, how can I conceptualise this? Is there a picture which can be of help to me, and indeed to others with whom I work? How can I hold to a concept of a communion of saints which will both work for people who believe in an 'afterlife' and hold dearly to the belief that they will be reunited with their loved ones in heaven, and bring comfort and reassurance to those who have no belief in a life after death, and no language to encapsulate their oneness with those who have gone before?

I suspect anthropologists can share insights with us from ancient tribal cultures, 'ancestor worship' and all the rest. But for me it has to be simpler than that. So I offer another picture, which I suppose, in one way or another, makes sense for me of all the rest.

It is a picture which comes from two sources. It arises firstly from the Ecumenical Institute, a Chicago-based church organisation I touched base with a number of years ago, whose task was to share insights for a modern day of Christian teaching. But it also derives from a vague recollection from Old Testament studies when I was in divinity college, so vague, indeed, that I fear the saints who were my professors and lecturers might wonder whether I learned anything at all at their feet!

Let me begin with this second source. I recall am image shared with us regarding the Prophets of the Old Testament. If I remember correctly, these Prophets were deemed to be in communion with God – from whence came their prophecies – so closely in communion that they somehow entered into the very dwelling place of God, into God's inner sanctum, and there communed with him and – and here is the point – with the saints and prophets who had gone before. Now, I may have got it wrong, but it was an image which made sense to me and which, right or wrong, has stuck with me ever since.

The Ecumenical Institute had this idea: in your head, in that inner part of your being, there is a table, big or small, and round that table sit people who matter to you, who influence you, who deeply affect your life. They may be alive or dead, they may be intimate contacts or people you have never met, they may be of greater or lesser importance. But because they matter to you, they are part of you, for ever at one with you, they are round your table – and so they are for you your communion of saints.

So, consciously or subconsciously, in specific or vague ways, sometimes without any particular knowledge that it is happening, you commune with them: you sit down round the table and talk and listen, and learn and absorb, from all those influences on you. And, like the prophets of old, you carry away what you need, of insight and clarity, of direction and decision.

Everyone has a table. Everyone has their saints. Everyone has their time of communion. Everyone is influenced.

My table? Well, the people in this book are there, as are my mother and father, and many people who have long since died. My wife and children are there, respected colleagues and trusted friends. Tom Paxton because of the insights from his songs and John Bell for similar reasons with his hymns have their place. My great heroes are there – St Peter, Martin Luther King and George MacLeod, among others. Living and dead, big and small, intimate and distant, these are my saints.

So I commune with them, still learning from what they have shared and share still. I am at one with them. And when those who are living pass from this life, they still have their place at my table; their influence does not diminish.

There are three parts of this personal image of the communion of saints which I utilise with people, particularly those who have been bereaved. The first is the idea that we are influenced by, and so we still learn from, the people who matter to us, even though they are dead, such has been the influence of a relationship with them on our lives. The second is that even unsaintly people can be our saints – sainthood is not about perfection! And the third is that in life and in death there is no distinction regarding their place at our table.

The first death I experienced in my close family circle was that of my grandfather, my mother's father, a cantankerous old man who had struggled in the final years of his life with advanced Parkinson's disease. Some weeks after he died, I went to visit my granny to see how she was coping. While I was there a neighbour took me aside and confided that she thought my granny was going mad, because she could hear her talking to herself in her house, and she knew it wasn't the TV or radio. I had a word with my granny, asking her why she was talking to herself. 'I've never talked to myself in my life, son,' she replied. 'So why are you talking when there's no one here?' I enquired. She looked at me as if I was daft. 'I'm talking to your grandpa, son,' she said. 'Grandpa?' I exclaimed. 'But grandpa's dead, granny.' 'I ken that fine, son,' the old lady continued – with a sympathetic smile that told me I had a lot yet to understand – 'but would you stop talking to someone who'd been your constant companion for over fifty years? I can't. So I talk to him, as if he were still sitting in his chair. The difference now is that I always get the last word and he can't start any arguments!'

The reassurance that she wasn't going mad came from her and not from me. But quite certainly my gran was still 'in communion' with this dominant figure round her table. There was nothing scary or mad or peculiar about it. For her it was a natural thing.

This is not to deny the reality of the death. It is not a syndrome that indicates that people are not prepared to accept the loss and are pretending their loved one is still there. It is, I believe, a natural affinity, a bond with the dead person which has its expression in this and other ways.

Meg was a widow with whom I worked in our bereavement service for some months. At the beginning of her grief, she couldn't even speak without breaking down in tears. But slowly, over the weeks and months, she found herself able to talk – about her husband, her teenage family, her struggles to cope, and the unfolding of her grief. I remember her saying through her tears in the early days, 'I feel Simon getting further and further away. I feel he and I are drifting apart, that we're no longer close. I find things in the house that mattered deeply to us both – a photograph, a gift, a cushion, a sweater – and I hold them close to me so that he might be close too.

But he isn't. He never is. I have lost him for ever.'

That pain of separation, and the finality of it, is very real in times of loss. And, of course, Meg is right – Simon is gone, for ever, and the separation is complete. But in time – and in the journey of sorrow this surely is the important factor – in time, a new closeness will emerge. I do not know whether Meg has yet found that – we have not been in contact since those early months – but my gut feeling is that she was getting there. And that gut feeling comes from what I have seen happen to others, and what I know of myself as I have dealt with my own losses. Of course, in physical terms, those who have influenced me have gone. But their influence – and a new understanding of their relationship with me, and the love and vitality that goes with it – most certainly has not.

I am not setting out in this chapter, or indeed in this book, to give a treatise on bereavement. But I am saying what I believe to be true, that the image of the table, used well, can explain what is happening to people and can be a strength to them in their understanding of questions about how the links remain and how the influence and the relationship continues.

The question, I suppose, is therefore, 'Who are the people round my table?' Who matters? Who remains when death comes? That, I believe, should make us look at the relationships which matter to us, and do it now.

In addition, there is this profoundly challenging thought. If I have people round my table, it is just possible – indeed, I hope it might be true – that there are people who have me sitting round their table along with their heroes and saints. Goodness! I hope, as Stevenson suggests, that I can, at least as far as I am able, 'behave mannerly' while I am there. And I hope that I might be an influence for someone, somewhere, which will continue after I die, unsaintly saint though I may be, so that in life and death my being, what I am and what I will continue to be, will go on being important.

'Bless 'em all, bless 'em all, the long and the short and the tall', runs the old song. And I suppose that is just what I mean in this business of defining our saints. Take wee Danny, for example. Danny had been a patient of ours for some time. He was a character – cheeky, quick-witted, good fun, sharp-tongued – and we all loved him, especially the nurses. Danny knew he was dying. He had seen other people die in his room, and he knew one day it would be his turn. After a particularly sad death of a young man he'd got to know well, Danny and I had a lengthy conversation. Yes he was sad, for he and Norman had become good friends. And, yes, he was deeply concerned for Norman's young wife. But he went further – this cocky wee man, with whom I'd never talked at a deep level, and who would never, as far as I knew, have considered himself even vaguely religious – and said this: 'Norman's just gone on ahead, Tom. He's just going to get there a wee bit before me. And I've asked him to keep my seat warm.' I knew exactly what he meant. We didn't need to talk about the details, about concepts of heaven, or the communion of saints, and the like. We just let his profound statement sit for a while. Then I smiled, and with tears in my eyes I said to Danny: 'When you've got your seat with Norman, will you keep a seat warm for me too?' 'Consider it done, son,' he replied with a wink. 'It would be no fun unless we were both there.'

The long and the short – and in this case the very short and cheeky Danny – and the tall all have their place. 'Good people, of every sort' as Oliver Goldsmith puts it, all giving ear to each other's song – and cheek, and advice, and guidance, and insights, and love, and much, much more besides. That's good enough for me! And I'm glad that this wee man is still round my table and, thank God, that he still has a place for me round his.

As I leave this image, let me offer this little postscript in the form of a question: 'Is it possible for fictional characters to have their place round my table?' I think it is. Can we not be affected, deeply stimulated and encouraged by the great heroes and lovers and actors of fiction? Of course we can. For are these characters not the product of the minds of those who see in their heads – round their own tables – that these characters are real and vibrant people? Let this table not be limited to what fits our restricted thinking and understanding. Let it be an abundant and stimulating place, full of life and colour and influence.

Yes, indeed, good people of every sort, and – quite remarkably, don't you think? – with you and me included.

My saints

'Tell them I was drum major for peace,' he said,
his ringing words touching the hearts of those who heard,
and touching mine
as they ring out again from printed page.
He's at my table,
and Martin Luther King and I talk of peace
and justice
and reconciliation,
and I am enlivened again.

'God loves you, son, and everything'll be OK,' she said,
often,
and much more besides.
The wisdom of years,
and the certainty of faith.
That's why wee granny's there –
her simplicity and love-in-action
give her an honoured place.

'When I get there, I'll keep your seat warm, son,' said Danny.
Who could doubt it, wee man?
That's my seat beside him there,
on his bed when he was dying,
and round the table now – and for always.
That's why you're there, wee Danny.
Even death itself couldn't separate us.

'To be a pilgrim,' he wrote.
And when hobgoblins and foul fiends
are vanquished,
am I not still encouraged by his pilgrimage
to be a pilgrim too?
John Bunyan –
did he know his faith would place him there
where he would always be,
where we could sing of pilgrimage together?

His music put him there,
the first time I heard it,
and often since,
as notes of beauty lifted me
from dull humanity to heights of wonder.
His music –
and others' too –
but Mozart has his place
to touch my soul
and make it truly sing.

And beauty, too,
gives others room,
and triumph,
invention
compassion
love
gives others their rightful place.

And when they made me laugh,
or tilted at windmills,
and shared their hugs
and offered their songs,
they became my people,
my guests,
my saints,
my communion.

These people …
Thy people …
Now my people, my saints …

Do I not for them have my honoured place?

The lesson from and the purpose of this chapter is quite simple – it is to help us to think about our own saints. Who are the people that matter who sit round our table? It is useful to try to pin that down, to think of who these people actually are and why they are important to us.

- So, take a big sheet of paper.

- Draw a circle or oval on it to represent your table.

- Put some seats round the table – smaller circles round the outside. (Don't make them too big at the start as you might find there are more saints in your life than you think!)

- Write the names of your saints in each circle, and as you do so think of why it is important that they are round your table. (Remember, they may be living or dead, real or fictional – it's their influence that matters.)

- If it is helpful, write alongside each name the reasons why they have their place.

- Keep adding to – or, indeed, taking away from – the seating arrangement as and when people's influence on you becomes more or less important.

- If you don't like the idea of a big sheet of paper, write a list of the names of your saints in your journal or diary and the reasons for your choice beside each name. This will serve the same purpose.

- And remember to give yourself a place. These saints are not much use to you unless you spend time with them round the table!

Seventeen

The picture gallery

Can I see another's woe, and not be in sorrow too?
Can I see another's grief, and not seek for kind relief?
William Blake: On Another's Sorrow

Why, this is not a drawing, but an inspiration!
Blake, of a painting by John Constable

Spirituality is on the agenda of our modern culture. Of that I am
certain. Consequently, rediscovery of spiritual care has never been
more needed. We all need to be helped to make sense of the struggles we face daily to be holistic in our care with limited time and
resources and little or no education in the whole area of spirituality.

One way of helping all of us to recognise the importance of
spirituality, and to keep spiritual care fully in the forefront of our
minds, is to move on from saying it is too nebulous to be defined
properly, and to become comfortable with images of what we are
working with which can give us a framework of understanding and
definition. This, I believe, is the beginning of the effectiveness of the
images in this picture gallery.

Many are fearful about a genuine attempt to understand spiritual
care and to enter into its meaning in practice because on the one hand
they don't know what to do, and on the other hand when they do feel
they know what to do they simply try too hard to get it right. Spiritual
care has loose ends! We cannot tie it up with red ribbon. But we have
to begin to be confident that what we do is good, and that what we do
actually works. And if you want it in religious terms, God makes sense
of things even when you can't!

I recall a scene from the film *The Shoes of the Fisherman*, in which

Anthony Quinn, who plays a dissident Russian priest who becomes Pope, ventures into the back streets of Rome from the security and grandeur of the Papal Palace. He finds himself with a doctor friend in the home of a dying man. There, dressed as a priest, he does the priestly thing and begins to say the Last Rites over the patient. He is stopped by the doctor who points to a Star of David on the wall and whispers: 'There are no Catholics here, Father, this is a Jewish household.' Quinn takes a step back and, after a moment's pause, places his hand over his eyes and begins to chant a Yiddish prayer. After a while the dying man's brother joins in the obviously familiar words, as do elderly women watching from the edge of the room. It is a moment of deep meaning and spirituality. There is a peace in the room. In time Quinn and the doctor take their leave. The dying man's brother says thank you. 'The dying is easy,' he sighs. 'It's the living that's hard.'

These people, as well as facing death were, even more importantly, facing a need for living. Yet in that place where living was supremely difficult, a Catholic priest – a Pope, indeed – offered a Hebrew prayer as a spiritual offering to the living in their need. It is not that we have to be all things to all people. (I confessed earlier that I know next to nothing of New Testament Greek. I confess now that I do not know a word of Hebrew!) But it is that we have surely to be responsive to needs as we find them, to enter into the painful living of those for whom we are called to care, to be in their spiritual search what they need us to be, and to believe that in this way peace will come and healing will take place.

A student on placement with me once described me as a 'soul watcher'. I'm happy with that, because the desert, the companionship, sharing the tears, helping people move between their two rooms are all about watching the soul, entering into the life and struggles of the person for whom you would seek to care. I know for certain that entering into their world gives a powerful signal about our care and the healing power of Love, and is infinitely more effective than any of us would even dare to believe.

None of us who work with dying people can fully understand the feelings of those who journey to death because we ourselves are not dying. There are, however, some clues we can pick up along the way which can be of use to us as we interpret the meaning of our own mortality, and which we can offer to those with whom we journey. Which one of us does not need to do some work in our messy attic before time runs out? Which one of us does not need to reinterpret the 'contract' and deal in a refreshing way with our relationship with our God? Which one of us does not need to finish our business before we die? Which of us does not need to look back and see things in their proper perspective and trust that, whatever the future holds, that which carried us forward in the past will hold us in the future too?

It is our task to help those who journey to death to find peace through working with these and other images, so that they, and we, can let go of life with some sense of rightness and purpose.

When we go further and work with bereaved people it is first and foremost our task to seek to understand what they are going through. It is no different, I believe, from our task with dying people as we seek to enter their world – desert, journey, attic or whatever, and work with them where they are. The pictures, therefore, of the river, the painting, the young child, the table and the rock face help me to do that, and at least to begin to understand.

A bereaved relative told me recently that the most hurtful thing that happened in the immediate post-bereavement period was to see a friend approaching him down the street of his village and cross over to the other side of the road to avoid talking to him. There is pain in that. So if we move towards the bereaved, the lost, the lonely and the vulnerable, with all our feelings of inadequacy and lack of the right thing to say, we offer healing for the pain. Simply by not avoiding the issue we give a powerful signal to those who need it most that all is not lost.

These expressions of care, and the attempt at an understanding, are the beginning of a healing process. It is an important help to those on the journey of grief. To see people move through grief to some capacity to live again is, as I have said already, enormously rewarding.

These words from John L. Bell sum it up for me.

Unsure, when what was bright turns dark
And life, it seems, has lost its way,
We question what we once believed
And fear that doubt has come to stay.
We sense the worm that gnaws within
Has withered willpower, weakened bones,
And wonder whether all that's left
Is stumbling blocks or stepping stones.

Where minds and bodies reel with pain
Which nervous smiles can never mask,
And hope is forced to face despair
And all the things it dared not ask;
Aware of weakness, guilt or shame,
The will gives out, the spirit groans,
And clutching at each straw we find
More stumbling blocks than stepping stones.

Where family life has lost its bliss
And silences endorse mistrust,
Or anger boils and tempers flare
As love comes under threat from lust;
Where people cannot take the strain
Of worklessness and endless loans,
What pattern will the future weave –
Just stumbling blocks, no stepping stones?

Where hearts that once held love are bare
And faith, in shreds, compounds the mess;
Where hymns and prayers no longer speak
And former friends no longer bless;
And when the church where some belonged
No more their loyalty enthrones,
The plea is made, 'If you are there,
Turn stumbling blocks to stepping stones!'

Ah, God, You with the Maker's eye,
Can tell if all that's feared is real,
And see if life is more than what
We suffer, dread, despise and feel.
If some by faith no longer stand
Nor hear the truth your voice intones,
Stretch out your hand to help your folk
From stumbling blocks to stepping stones.

Yes, stepping stones can come from stumbling blocks. Wholeness can come from brokenness. New beginnings can come from the darkness of death. (I have never been quite sure why Marie Cure Cancer Care chose the daffodil as their emblem. But as the daffodil is one of the most potent symbols of new life in the spring, breaking through from the darkness and deadness of the winter earth, perhaps the meaning is not too hard to understand.)

While I was preparing this final chapter, I had an important discussion with a young widow. Three months after her husband's death she had got stuck, and needed again to go over the events around his death to try to understand what had happened, whether she could have done anything differently, if she had let him down, and a number of other issues. I met her with one of our doctors, and from a medical and an emotional perspective we took time to help her review things, and as we did so we could feel her responding to what we were offering.

Towards the conclusion of our discussions the doctor said, 'It's as if you've gone into a siding. That's OK, because you've needed to stop and look at some things. All we are doing is taking time with you there, looking at what needs to be looked at, and helping you to get ready to start again. You'll be ready in your own time to come out of the siding and restart the journey.'

Another picture, and one I'd not thought of using before. So I continued, 'Yes, and that's fine. But when you back out of the siding and start to go forward again, if you haven't got things sorted properly, you'll go full steam straight back into the siding! So, once you've backed out, before you start getting up steam to recommence the journey, you have to make a decision, to change the points on the track to make sure you're heading up the main line again. We can do our bit, but you have to do yours too. And once you have made the conscious choice to change the points, then you will be ready to go again.'

The doctor smiled. So did the young widow. And another image was doing its work once more.

In his book *Companions on the Inner Way*, Father Morton Kelsey writes: 'Walking with others on their spiritual pilgrimages is an art like painting or sculpture or poetry. In painting there are many things we need to learn. Great artists usually learn from others.'

I have many things still to learn about my pictures — how to use them, to develop them, to add to them — but as I walk with others on their spiritual pilgrimages I hope that they too can learn from me, and that you have learned a little from the pictures in this gallery. Perhaps they can even become signposts — on the journey of life and beyond!

In writing this book, I have continued to reflect on my own pictures and how they have been composed. And as I learn about my own techniques, I also need to continue to learn from others, to share their discoveries, to see further advances in an understanding of spiritual care.

We are a long way from perfection. But we have begun the process. The canvasses have been prepared. The first paintings have been completed. The gallery is open. The work has begun.

Thank you

Thank you
for the times you came to me
when I least expected it –
in the helpful image,
the comforting word,
the holy moment,
when what we shared together
became your sacrament
of grace and love.

Thank you
for the people you sent
when I needed them most –
for the insight,
the touch,
the smile,
that showed what God was like

Thank you
for the beauty you gave
when life was ugly
and distorted with pain and sorrow –
for a peaceful death,
a loving family,

a fresh start,
a new day,
when there was the beauty of hope again,
for eternity,
for time,
and for now.

Thank you
for the wonder you shared –
when I thought I knew you
or could explain you
or offer you to others,
and learned again
of mystery
and depth
and your unfathomable being,
gathering everything up –
and me! –
in love
for you.

Thank you
for life,
for being,
for love,
for you,
for me.

Thank you
for this.

References and copyright acknowledgements

Pages 11–12
Pandora's Box
Words and music by Tom Paxton
Copyright © 1977 Pax Music (ASCAP) and Dream Works Songs (ASCAP)
Worldwide rights for Pax Music and Dream Works Songs administered by
Cherry Lane Music Company, Inc. International Copyright Secured. All
Rights Reserved.

Pages 32–33
My Skies
Copyright © James Keelaghan, from the album *My Skies*, published by Red
Bird/Green Linnet, CLGD 2112, 1993

Page 41
Extract from *Community and Growth* by Jean Vanier; copyright © Jean
Vanier 1979. Published by Paulist Press, Mahwah, NJ, USA. Used with
permission of Paulist Press: www.paulistpress.com

Page 44 & 46
Extracts taken from *Sharing the Darkness* by Sheila Cassidy, published and
copyright © 1988 by Darton Longman and Todd Ltd, and used by permission of the publishers.

Page 48
Who is There to Understand?
Copyright © John L. Bell & Graham Maule, The Iona Community, Glas-
gow, 1996. Reproduced from *When Grief is Raw*, published by Wild Goose
Publications, 1997.

Page 55
Extract from the writing of Harold Kushner. *When Bad Things Happen to
Good People*, by Harold Kushner, published 2000, Pan Books, USA.

Page 58
Extract from *The Go-Between God* by John V. Taylor, published by SCM Press, 1972.

Page 71
Towards Calmer Waters
Extract (anonymous) from *Words for Worship*, edited and compiled by Christopher Campling and Michael Davis, published by Edward Arnold, 1969.

Pages 101 & 102
Extracts from *The Heart of Enlightenment* by Anthony de Mello, published by Fount Paperbacks (now part of HarperCollins Publishers Ltd), 1989.

Page 193
Extract from *Strange Places, Questionable People* by John Simpson, published by Macmillan Publishers, 1998.

Pages 209–10
Stumbling Blocks to Stepping Stones
Copyright © John L. Bell & Graham Maule, Iona Community, 1989
Reproduced from *Love From Below*, published by Wild Goose Publications, 1989, 1992.

Page 211
Extract from Companions on the *Inner Way*, by Morton Kelsey, published by the Crossroad Publishing Company, NY, 1983.

All biblical quotations are from the *Good News Bible*, published by The Bible Societies/HarperCollins Publishers Ltd UK © American Bible Society, 1966, 1971, 1976, 1992.

Index of exercises, prayers and reflections

WHEN GRIEF IS RAW
Songs for times of sorrow and bereavement
John L. Bell & Graham Maule

Specifically designed for congregational use, this songbook from the innovative and popular Wild Goose Resource Group contains 25 songs for times of sorrow and loss. The songs have straightforward arrangements, either four-part harmony or with simple piano accompaniment.

Pbk · 0 947988 91 2 · £8.99

PRAYING FOR THE DAWN
A resource book for the ministry of healing
Ruth Burgess & Kathy Galloway (eds)

A compilation of material, with a strong emphasis on liturgies and resources for healing services. Aspects of healing addressed include

The Church's healing ministry ● The Iona Community service of prayers for healing ● Justice as healing ● The National Health Service and the health of the nation ● The healing of Northern Ireland ● The memory of brokenness ● To die healed ● The laying on of hands

Some of the liturgies featured:
A service of prayers for healing and the laying on of hands ● Keeping the Earth beautiful: a service of creation and healing for all ages ● An order of prayer for people with chronic illness ● For those facing serious illness ● Service for all souls ● Liturgy for carers

Includes a section of worship resources – prayers, responses, litanies, poems, meditations and blessings.

Pbk · 1 901557 26 X · £10.99

Prayers and Ideas for Healing Services
Ian Cowie

The author draws on his decades of experience to provide a complete guide to healing ministry which combines sound practical advice with conviction, refreshing realism and compassion. Also included are suggested orders of service, prayers for blessing and healing, prayers of guided silence for approach, confession, intercession, invocation, healing of relationships, etc.

Pbk · 0 947988 72 6 · £7.99

Love From Below
Songbook/CD/cassette from the Wild Goose Worship Group
John L. Bell & Graham Maule

Songs of discipleship and the Church's sacraments and seasons including:

A touching place ● *Listen Lord* ● *Shout for joy* ● *Come Lord and be our guest* ● *Blessed are you poor* ● *Stumbling blocks to stepping stones* ● *Kyrie Sanctus and Benedictus/Agnus Dei (Ninian setting)*

The book contains 62 songs and the CD/cassette 16

Songbook · *0 947988 34 3 · £8.99* **Cassette** · *0 947988 63 7 · £8.50* **CD** · *1 901557 46 4 · £14.99*

Jesus' Healing Works ... and Ours
Ian Cowie

Possibly the first book to cover every single healing miracle of the New Testament, including those of the apostles. Ian Cowie, in a very direct and informative way, re-translates the original Greek of the gospels and sheds new light on what the miracles of Jesus actually were and what they mean for us.

Pbk · 1 901557 27 8 · £9.99

The Iona Community

The Iona Community, founded in 1938 by the Revd George MacLeod, then a parish minister in Glasgow, is an ecumenical Christian community committed to seeking new ways of living the Gospel in today's world. Initially working to restore part of the medieval abbey on Iona, the Community today remains committed to 'rebuilding the common life' through working for social and political change, striving for the renewal of the church with an ecumenical emphasis, and exploring new, more inclusive approaches to worship, all based on an integrated understanding of spirituality.

The Community now has over 240 Members, about 1500 Associate Members and around 1500 Friends. The Members – women and men from many denominations and backgrounds (lay and ordained), living throughout Britain with a few overseas – are committed to a fivefold Rule of devotional discipline, sharing and accounting for use of time and money, regular meeting, and action for justice and peace.

At the Community's three residential centres – the Abbey and the MacLeod Centre on Iona, and Camas Adventure Camp on the Ross of Mull – guests are welcomed from March to October and over Christmas. Hospitality is provided for over 110 people, along with a unique opportunity, usually through week-long programmes, to extend horizons and forge relationships through sharing an experience of the common life in worship, work, discussion and relaxation. The Community's shop on Iona, just outside the Abbey grounds, carries an attractive range of books and craft goods.

The Community's administrative headquarters are in Glasgow, which also serves as a base for its work with young people, the Wild Goose Resource Group working in the field of worship, a bi-monthly magazine, Coracle, and a publishing house, Wild Goose Publications.

For information on the Iona Community contact:
The Iona Community
Pearce Institute
840 Govan Road
Glasgow G51 3UU, UK
Phone: 0141 445 4561
e-mail: ionacomm@gla.iona.org.uk   web: www.iona.org.uk